Hormones and Cell Regulation (n° 14)

Hormones et Régulation Cellulaire (n° 14)

Colloques **INSERM**
ISSN 0768-3154

Other *Colloques* published as co-editions by John Libbey Eurotext and INSERM

133 Cardiovascular and Respiratory Physiology in the Fetus and Neonate. *Physiologie Cardiovasculaire et Respiratoire du Fœtus et du Nouveau-né.*
Scientific Committee : P. Karlberg,
A. Minkowski, W. Oh and L. Stern;
Managing Editor : M. Monset-Couchard.
ISBN : John Libbey Eurotext 0 86196 125 0
INSERM 2 85598 340 1

134 Porphyrins and Porphyrias. *Porphyrines et Porphyries.*
Edited by Y. Nordmann.
ISBN : John Libbey Eurotext 0 86196 087 4
INSERM 2 85598 281 2

137 Neo-Adjuvant Chemotherapy. *Chimiothérapie Néo-Adjuvante.*
Edited by C. Jacquillat, M. Weil and D. Khayat.
ISBN : John Libbey Eurotext 0 86196 125 0
INSERM 2 85598 340 1

139 Hormones and Cell Regulation (10th European Symposium). *Hormones et Régulation Cellulaire (10ᵉ Symposium Européen).*
Edited by J. Nunez, J.E. Dumont and R. J.B. King.
ISBN : John Libbey Eurotext 0 86196 125 0X
INSERM 2 85598 340 1

147 Modern Trends in Aging Research. *Nouvelles Perspectives de la Recherche sur le Vieillissement.*
Edited by Y. Courtois, B. Faucheux, B. Forette, D.L. Knook and J.A. Tréton.
ISBN : John Libbey Eurotext 0 86196 126 0X
INSERM 2 85598 340 1

149 Binding Proteins of Steroid Hormones. *Protéines de liaison des Hormones Stéroïdes.*
Edited by M.G. Forest and M. Pugeat.
ISBN : John Libbey Eurotext 0 86196 125 0
INSERM 2 85598 340 1X

151 Control and Management of Parturition. *La Maîtrise de la Parturition.*
Edited by C. Sureau, P. Blot, D. Cabrol, F. Cavaillé and G. Germain.
ISBN : John Libbey Eurotext 0 86196 125 0
INSERM 2 85598 340 1

Suite page 123

II

Hormones and Cell Regulation

Hormones et Régulation Cellulaire

Proceedings of the 14th INSERM European Symposium on Hormones
and Cell Regulation, held at Mont Sainte-Odile (France), September
25-28, 1989

Sponsored by the Institut National de la Santé
et de la Recherche Médicale (INSERM)

Edited by

J. Nunez
J.E. Dumont

LES EDITIONS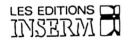
INSERM

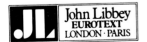 John Libbey
EUROTEXT
LONDON · PARIS

III

British Library Cataloguing in Publication Data
INSERM European Symposium on Hormones and
   Cell Regulation (*14th, 1989, Sainte-Odile, France*)
   Hormones and cell regulation
   1. Organisms. Cells. Metabolism. Regulation.
   Role of Hormones
   I. Title. II. Nunez, J. (Jacques), *1927*
   III Dumont, J.E. (Jacques E.), *1931*
   IV. Séries
   574.87'61
ISBN 0-86196-229-X

First published in 1989 by

John Libbey Eurotext Ltd
6 rue Blanche, 92120 Montrouge, France. (1) 47 35 85 52
ISBN 0 86196 229-X

John Libbey & Company Ltd
13 Smiths Yard, Summerley Street, London SW18 4HR,
England.
(1) 947 27 77

**Institut National de la Santé et de la Recherche
Médicale**
101 rue de Tolbiac, 75654 Paris Cedex 13, France.
(1) 45 84 14 41
ISBN 2 85598 400 9

ISSN 0768-3154

Proceedings of the annual European Symposia on **Hormones and Cell Regulation** held every autumn since 1976 have been published by Elsevier Biomedical Press in a series co-edited by INSERM [*] from Volume 1 to Volume 9.

The 10th Symposium held in 1985 and the next ones are now published as co-editions by John Libbey Eurotext and INSERM in the series "Colloques INSERM" (Vol. 139, Vol. 153, Vol. 165, Vol. 176, Vol. 198).

[*] except Vol. 7 published by Elsevier

Préface

Quatorze ans sont passés depuis qu'un petit groupe de scientifiques a ressenti le besoin d'organiser en Europe une réunion annuelle sur le thème général «Hormones et régulation cellulaire». A l'époque, la découverte des récepteurs et des systèmes cyclasiques d'amplification membranaire du signal hormonal ouvrait de multiples perspectives expérimentales qui se sont vérifiées par la suite. En effet, ces modèles ont permis non seulement de comprendre le mécanisme d'action de nombreuses hormones mais ils se sont révélés opérationnels dans de nombreux autres domaines : action de nombreux neuromédiateurs, régulation de l'activité des canaux ioniques, mécanisme de la vision et de l'olfaction, activation du système immunitaire, etc. De ce fait, le titre même du colloque apparaît dépassé, la notion beaucoup plus générale de signal d'information se substituant progressivement à celle d'hormone. Ainsi, aux systèmes cyclasiques d'amplification de la première période, s'ajoutaient divers types de messagers lipidiques, notamment les phosphoinositides et les prostaglandines, des ions tels le calcium et, enfin, toute une classe de molécules d'information regroupées sous la dénomination de facteurs de croissance mais qui, en définitive, pourraient être considérées comme des hormones.

La seconde révolution conceptuelle est intervenue lorsque l'on a commencé à comprendre que la distinction classique entre actions rapides et modulatrices (phasiques) de ces divers facteurs de signalisation et effets lents (trophiques) des mêmes molécules n'était, en grande partie, que le reflet de l'imperfection de nos connaissances. Le domaine primitivement couvert par le colloque s'est ainsi élargi progressivement aux recherches sur la régulation de l'expression génique, aux oncogènes et antioncogènes, etc. En ce qui concerne les oncogènes, par exemple, on a rapidement réalisé que beaucoup d'entre eux sont soit des récepteurs hormonaux ou des facteurs de croissance, soit des protéines impliquées, dans la membrane ou le génome, dans la transduction des divers signaux d'information. Des relations inattendues apparaissent ainsi entre l'endocrinologie et les mécanismes de la transformation virale. Une jonction entre l'endocrinologie *stricto sensu,* la génétique moléculaire, la neurobiologie, l'embryologie et la différenciation, la pathologie moléculaire, l'immunologie, etc. pouvait ainsi intervenir. On trouvera dans le programme de cette année une ou plusieurs conférences portant sur ces diverses thématiques.

Les colloques que nous avons organisés chaque année sont ainsi le reflet de cette évolution. Ils répondent de ce fait à l'un des objectifs de départ : celui de proposer à l'audience une vision à la fois précise et diversifiée des mécanismes de régulation cellulaire et intercellulaire en voie d'exploration dans divers systèmes. Le programme de cette année n'échappe pas, nous l'espérons du moins, à cette règle. Conçu dans ses grandes lignes par un Comité Scientifique composé de chercheurs européens, indépendants dans le choix des thèmes et des conférenciers, et mis en œuvre par un Secrétaire Scientifique chaque année différent, le colloque bénéficie du soutien très actif de l'INSERM tant sur le plan financier qu'administratif. Depuis sa fondation, plus de 1 500 chercheurs y ont participé comme auditeurs et aussi comme présentateurs de nombreux travaux affichés. La dimension européenne du colloque s'affirme ainsi de plus en plus et devrait s'amplifier dans les années à venir.

J. Nunez

Foreword

The 14th European Symposium on Hormones and Cell Regulation is focused on two complementary areas. The first area concerns gene regulation including the control of protooncogenes and antioncogenes. The studies presented start from the fundamental problems of the control of gene expression and considering the modulation of protooncogenes and antioncogenes in cell proliferation, end up with the role of oncogenes in cell transformation. The second area is the relation of the cell with its environment through ionic channels and receptors for extracellular signals. In these fields also the genes of the proteins are cloned or about to be cloned and the sequences will give us crucial information on their function. A general conference on the control of cells of the immune system is also programmed.

The speakers have been chosen in Europe when it was possible, in the US or elsewhere when it was necessary. Their group gives a good representation of the Europe of Science. In general, we also tried to recruit scientists who still work "at the bench" and fully conversant with their methodology, rather than the classical travelling speakers who make the congress circuit.

A selection of posters will be presented orally in plenary session.

It is hoped that the 14th Symposium will be as successful as the previous ones.

J.E. Dumont
Brussels

The Conference was sponsored by INSERM, Paris, France.

Avant-propos

Le 14ᵉ Symposium Européen sur les Hormones et la Régulation Cellulaire a été focalisé sur deux domaines complémentaires. Le premier concerne la régulation des gènes et, notamment, des protooncogènes et antioncogènes. Les travaux présentés partent des problèmes fondamentaux sur le contrôle de l'expression génique pour aboutir à la modulation des protooncogènes dans la croissance cellulaire et des oncogènes et protooncogènes dans la transformation cancéreuse. Le second concerne le rapport de la cellule avec son milieu ambiant par l'intermédiaire de canaux ioniques et de récepteurs. Dans ces domaines aussi, des gènes de protéines sont clonés ou en voie de clonage, et les séquences nous donneront des renseignements cruciaux sur leur fonction. Une conférence générale est consacrée au contrôle, dans les cellules, du système immunitaire.

Les orateurs ont été choisis en Europe quand cela était possible, aux Etats-Unis ou dans d'autres pays quand cela était nécessaire. Leur groupe donne une bonne représentation de l'Europe de la Science. En général, nous avons tenté de recruter des scientifiques travaillant encore au laboratoire et au fait de leur méthodologie plutôt que les orateurs voyageurs que l'on retrouve dans tous les congrès.

Par ailleurs, une sélection de posters sera présentée, oralement, en session plénière.

Nous espérons que le 14ᵉ Symposium sera digne de ses prédécesseurs.

J.E. Dumont
Bruxelles

La conférence était organisée avec le soutien de l'INSERM, Paris, France.

List and address of organizers

Liste et adresse des organisateurs

Carafoli E., Laboratorium für Biochemie, ETH-Zentrum, CH-8092 Zurich, Switzerland.

Dentom R.M., Department of Biochemistry, School of Medical Sciences, University of Bristol, Bristol, BS8 1TD, UK.

Dumont J.E., Université Libre de Bruxelles, IRIBHN, Faculté de Médecine, Campus Hôpital Erasme, Bât C, Route de Lennik, 808, B-1070 Brussels, Belgium.

Hamprecht B., Physiologisch-Chemisches Institut, Universität Tübingen, Hoppe-Seyler-Strasse 4, 7400 Tübingen 1, Federal Republic of Germany.

King R., Imperial Cancer Research Fund Labs, Hormone Biochemistry Department, PO Box 123, Lincoln's Inn Fields, London, WC2A 3PX, UK.

Moolenaar W.H., Hubrecht Laboratory, Uppsala Laan 8, 3584 CT Utrecht, The Netherlands.

Morel F., Collège de France, Laboratoire de Physiologie Cellulaire, 11, place Marcelin Berthelot, 75231 Paris Cedex 05, France.

Nunez J., INSERM U 282, Hôpital Henri-Mondor, 94010 Créteil, France.

Schultz G., Institut für Pharmakologie, Freie Universität Berlin, Thielallee 69/73, D-1000 Berlin 33, Federal Republic of Germany.

Van der Molen H., Department of Biochemistry II, Erasmus Universitcit Rotterdam, 3000 Rotterdam, The Netherlands.

List and address of speakers
Liste et adresse des orateurs

Ashcroft S.J.H., Nuffield Dept. of Clinical Biochemistry, University of Oxford, John Radcliffe Hospital, Headington, Oxford OX39DU, UK.

Bernards R., Dept of Molecular Genetics, Massachusetts General Hospital East, 149, 13th Street, Charlestown, MA 02129, USA.

Boshart M., Deutsches Krebsforshungszentrum, Institut für Zell-und Tumorbiologie, Im Neuenheimer Feld, 280, D-6900 Heidelberg, Federal Republic of Germany.

Chinkers M., Department of Physiology, Vanderbilt University, School of Medicine, Nashville, Tenn 37232, USA.

Fahrenholz F., Max-Planck-Institut für Biophysik, Kennedy-Allee, 70, 6000 Frankfurt 70, Federal Republic of Germany.

Frelin C., Centre de Biochimie CNRS, Université de Nice, Parc Valrose, 06034 Nice Cedex, France.

Henley J.M., MRC Molecular Neurobiology Unit, University of Cambridge, Medical School, Hills Road, Cambridge CB2 2QH, UK.

Mallat M., INSERM U.114, Collège de France, 11, Place Marcelin-Berthelot, 75231 Paris Cedex 05, France.

Rusconi S., Institut für Molekularbiologie II der Universität Zurich, Hönggerberg, CH-8093 Zurich, Switzerland.

Salomon Y., Department of Hormone Research, The Weizmann Institute of Science, Rehovot 76100, Israel.

Scholer H., Department of Molecular Cell Biology Max-Planck-Institut für, Biophysikalische Chemie, Postfach 28 41, D-3400 Gotttingen, Federal Republic of Germany.

Serrano R., European Molecular Biology Lab., Postfach 10.2209, Meyerhofstrasse, 1, D-6900 Heidelberg, Federal Republic of Germany.

Simpson E.R., Cecil H. & Ida Green Center, 5323 Harry Hines Bld, Dallas, TX 75235-9051, USA.

Strehler E.E., Laboratorium für Biochemie, ETH-Zentrum, CH-8092 Zurich, Switzerland.

Theze J., Immunogénétique Cellulaire, Institut Pasteur, 25, rue du Dr. Roux, 75015 Paris, France.

Van Haastert P.M., Zoölogisch Laboratorium, Kaiserstraat 63, P.O. Box 9516, 2300 Ra Leiden, The Netherlands.

Vassart G., Institut de Recherche Interdisciplinaire, Faculté de Médecine, Université Libre de Bruxelles, 808 route de Lennik, B-1070 Brussels, Belgium.

Velu T.J., Laboratory of Cellular Oncology, Bldg 37, Room 1B26, National Cancer Institute NIH, Bethesda, MD 20892, USA.

Wasylyk B., INSERM U.184, Institut de Chimie Biologique, Faculté de Médecine, 11, rue Humann, 67085 Strasbourg Cedex, France.

Contents
Sommaire

REGULATION OF GENE EXPRESSION
RÉGULATION DE L'EXPRESSION GÉNIQUE

GROWTH FACTORS
FACTEURS DE CROISSANCE

CONTROL MECHANISMS IN OTHER SYSTEMS
MÉCANISMES DE CONTRÔLE DANS D'AUTRES SYSTÈMES

Surface receptors and cyclases

Récepteurs de surface et cyclases

Hormones and Cell Regulation. N° 14, Eds J. Nunez, J.E. Dumont. Colloque INSERM/J. Libbey Eurotext Ltd. © 1989. Vol. 198, pp. 3-6

Guanylate cyclase as a cell surface receptor

Michael Chinkers

Department of Pharmacology and the Howard Hughes Medical Institute, 702 Light Hall, Vanderbilt University Medical Center, Nashville, TN 37232-0295 USA

The enzyme guanylate cyclase exists in several molecular forms: an integral membrane protein, a heterodimeric protein located in the cytosol, and a cytoskeletal protein. In recent studies describing a new mechanism for signal transduction, the membrane form of guanylate cyclase has been implicated as a receptor for egg peptides from sea urchins and for atrial peptides from vertebrates. The observations that initially led to this hypothesis, and the recombinant DNA approaches used to confirm it, are described here. In the model that has emerged, binding of a peptide ligand to a guanylate cyclase/receptor on the surface of a target cell stimulates intracellular formation of cGMP, which then acts as a second messenger. Important sites of regulation by cGMP include ion channels, cGMP-dependent protein kinase, and cyclic nucleotide phosphodiesterase.

ACTIVATION OF SPERM MEMBRANE GUANYLATE CYCLASE BY SEA URCHIN EGG PEPTIDES

In the late 1970's, it was observed that medium conditioned by sea urchin eggs contained low molecular weight substances that activated the respiration and motility of sea urchin spermatozoa (reviewed in Garbers, 1988). The substances were purified from a variety of echinoderms and shown to be small, species-specific peptides; examples are speract (GFDLNGGGVG, from the sea urchin Strongylocentrotus purpuratus) and resact (CVTGAPGCVGGGRL-NH$_2$, from the sea urchin Arbacia punctulata). The effects of the egg peptides on spermatozoa were presumed to enhance fertilization. Both speract and resact bound with high affinity and in a species-specific manner to receptors present on the sperm cell surface. One of the initial responses to peptide binding was activation of a membrane form of guanylate cyclase, with resultant elevations of intracellular cGMP concentrations.

MEMBRANE GUANYLATE CYCLASE AS AN EGG PEPTIDE RECEPTOR

The inability to solubilize the egg peptide receptors in active form prevented their purification. However, crosslinking studies implicated a membrane form of guanylate cyclase as the resact receptor of A. punctulata spermatozoa. Radiolabeled resact was specifically crosslinked to a 160K protein identified as guanylate cyclase based on the following evidence (Shimomura, Dangott, & Garbers, 1986): (1) its apparent molecular weight; (2) a characteristic shift in apparent molecular weight induced by treatment of spermatozoa with ammonium chloride; and (3) its reactivity with antibodies to guanylate cyclase. In contrast, radiolabeled speract was specifically crosslinked to a 77K protein, unrelated to guanylate cyclase, on the surface of S. purpuratus spermatozoa (Dangott & Garbers, 1984; Dangott et al., 1989). This result was unexpected, given the similar

3

structures and physiological effects of egg peptides in both species. One interpretation was that guanylate cyclase and the 77K protein were closely apposed in the membrane, such that bound peptide might crosslink to either protein, depending on species differences in the accessibility of reactive side chains. Thus, the data were consistent with two possibilities: guanylate cyclase as a receptor for egg peptides, or guanylate cyclase as a protein closely associated with the receptor.

ACTIVATION OF MEMBRANE GUANYLATE CYCLASE BY ATRIAL NATRIURETIC PEPTIDES

At approximately the same time that the above studies were implicating a membrane form of guanylate cyclase as an egg peptide receptor, studies were being conducted to elucidate the mechanism of action of atrial natriuretic peptide (ANP) (see Inagami, 1989, for review). This polypeptide, synthesized in vertebrate cardiac atria, was shown to be released into the bloodstream in response to elevated central blood pressure, and to lower blood pressure by inducing natriuresis, diuresis, and vasodilation, as well as by inhibiting secretion of aldosterone, renin, and vasopressin. ANP, though unrelated to the egg peptides in primary structure or biological function, seemed to act through similar biochemical mechanisms. ANP was shown to bind with high affinity to receptors on the surface of target cells, and to induce rapid increases in intracellular cGMP concentrations by activating a membrane form of guanylate cyclase. cGMP was presumed to act as a second messenger for ANP, since many, though not all, effects of the hormone could be mimicked by cGMP.

MEMBRANE GUANYLATE CYCLASE AS AN ANP RECEPTOR

Crosslinking studies using radiolabeled ANP identified two receptors on the surface of target cells; both were purified to near-homogeneity (reviewed by Inagami, 1989). The low molecular weight (65K) receptor was apparently not coupled to cGMP increases, although disagreement exists on this point (Ishido et al., 1989). The function of the low molecular weight receptor was postulated to be the clearance of excess ANP from the circulation, and it was designated the ANP C-receptor (Maack et al., 1987). The ANP C-receptor consists of an extracellular binding domain, a single transmembrane domain, and a very small cytoplasmic domain (Fuller et al., 1988). The high molecular weight (130K) ANP receptor was shown to be coupled to cGMP increases (Leitman et al., 1986), and copurified extensively with guanylate cyclase activity. In some highly purified preparations, specific ANP binding activity approached the theoretical maximum, and guanylate cyclase activity was similar to that of homogeneous guanylate cyclase purified from sea urchin sperm membranes. These data suggested that both ANP-binding and guanylate cyclase activities resided in the same molecule, i.e. that a membrane form of guanylate cyclase was an ANP receptor. However, the very low quantities of purified ANP receptor obtained made demonstrations of homogeneity impossible, leaving open the possibility that ANP-binding and guanylate cyclase activities resided in separate but tightly associated molecules. In addition, the inability of ANP to activate guanylate cyclase in purified receptor preparations argued against both activities being present in the same protein.

ISOLATION OF A cDNA ENCODING A SEA URCHIN MEMBRANE GUANYLATE CYCLASE

The above data suggested the existence of receptors having intrinsic ligand-activated guanylate cyclase activity, but did not exclude the possibility that guanylate cyclase was merely closely associated with the actual binding proteins. In order to obtain a definitive answer to this question, the approach taken was to isolate cDNA clones encoding membrane guanylate cyclases, express them in cultured cells, and determine whether the proteins they encoded contained both guanylate cyclase and peptide binding activies. The high abundance of the membrane form of guanylate cyclase in sea urchin spermatozoa made this a logical starting point. Peptide sequences from the purified A. punctulata sperm membrane guanylate cyclase were used to design partially degenerate oligonucleotide probes, which, in turn, were used to screen an A. punctulata testis cDNA library (Singh et al., 1988).

4

cDNA clones were isolated that encoded a transmembrane protein identified as guanylate cyclase based on the following criteria: (1) all of the peptide sequences determined from the purified guanylate cyclase were present in the deduced amino acid sequence; (2) antisera to a peptide from the deduced amino acid sequence immunoprecipitated guanylate cyclase activity from A. punctulata sperm extracts; (3) amino acid sequences were conserved between this clone and a subunit of a bovine soluble guanylate cyclase (Singh et al., 1988).

Analysis of the deduced amino acid sequence of the A. punctulata guanylate cyclase predicted an amino-terminal signal sequence followed by a 478-residue extracellular domain, a single transmembrane domain, and a 459-residue intracellular domain. Proximal to the plasma membrane, the majority of the intracellular sequences consisted of a protein kinase-like domain, followed by a short region (about 60 amino acids) having homology to a subunit of a soluble guanylate cyclase (Koesling et al., 1988, Nakane et al., 1988). Because the similarity to soluble guanylate cyclase was so limited, and might not involve catalytic sequences, based on expression studies, it was tentatively suggested that GTP binding might occur in the protein kinase-like domain (Singh et al., 1988; Nakane et al., 1988). We have not yet detected protein kinase activity in sea urchin guanylate cyclase preparations.

ISOLATION OF A cDNA ENCODING A FUNCTIONAL GUANYLATE CYCLASE/ANP RECEPTOR

Screening of human cDNA libraries using the A. punctulata clone, under conditions of low stringency, led to the isolation of a partial-length human guanylate cyclase clone, which was used as a probe to isolate a full-length cDNA encoding a membrane guanylate cyclase from rat brain (Chinkers et al., 1989). The amino acid sequence deduced from the rat brain cDNA was generally similar to the sea urchin sequence described above, although the extracellular domains were divergent; the extracellular domain of the rat guanylate cyclase was highly homologous to the ANP C-receptor. Another difference was found in the intracellular domain: the sequences distal (carboxyl) to the protein kinase-like domain showed more extensive homology with the soluble guanylate cyclase (>200 amino acids), and with a region of the yeast adenylate cyclase known to be involved in catalysis (Chinkers et al., 1989; Kataoka et al., 1985). Since this large region of cyclase homology was also subsequently found in the membrane guanylate cyclase from the sea urchin S. purpuratus (Thorpe and Garbers, 1989), and is more highly conserved than the protein kinase-like domain, it seems likely that this is the guanylate cyclase catalytic domain; the published sequence of the A. punctulata enzyme could potentially be in error in this region.

Expression of the rat brain guanylate cyclase cDNA in cultured mammalian cells led to large increases in membrane-associated guanylate cyclase activity, which could be stimulated by ANP. This confirmed that the clone encoded a membrane guanylate cyclase. In addition, cells transfected with the guanylate cyclase cDNA bound approximately nine-fold more radiolabeled ANP than control cells. This demonstrated that a membrane guanylate cyclase was an ANP receptor. The binding characteristics of the recombinant guanylate cyclase/ANP receptor were similar to those reported for the receptor isolated from tissues, as was its apparent molecular weight determined by crosslinking experiments. Similar results were subsequently obtained when the partial-length human cDNA clone used to screen the rat library was ligated to appropriate 5' genomic sequences to yield a hybrid cDNA/genomic clone containing the complete coding region for a human guanylate cyclase/ANP receptor (Lowe et al., 1989).

SUMMARY AND PERSPECTIVES

The discovery that a recombinant membrane guanylate cyclase was an ANP receptor demonstrates the existence of a new receptor family. Members of this family contain an extracellular ligand-binding domain, a single putative transmembrane domain, a protein kinase-like domain, and a guanylate cyclase domain. The ability of the ANP receptor to produce cGMP in response to ligand binding contrasts with the more indirect hormonal regulation of cAMP production, in which receptors activate G proteins that modulate adenylate cyclase activity (Gilman, 1987). Current research is aimed at identifying and characterizing other members of the guanylate cyclase receptor family and the ligands to which they bind, and at defining structure/function relationships and mechanisms of regulation of the cloned ANP receptor. In addition to the potential clinical significance of studies using a cloned ANP receptor, the identification of this new receptor family opens a new area of research in cell biology.

REFERENCES

Chinkers, M., Garbers, D.L., Chang, M.-S., Lowe, D.G., Chin, H., Goeddel, D.G., and Schulz, S. (1989): A membrane form of guanylate cyclase is an atrial natriuretic peptide receptor. Nature 338, 78-83.

Dangott, L.J., and Garbers, D.L. (1984): Identification and partial characterization of the receptor for speract. J. Biol. Chem. 259, 13712-13716.

Dangott, L.J., Jordan, J.E., Bellet, R.A., and Garbers, D.L. (1989): Cloning of the mRNA for the protein that crosslinks to the egg peptide speract. Proc. Natl. Acad. Sci. U.S.A. 86, 2128-2132.

Fuller, F., Porter, J.G., Arfsten, A.E., Miller, J., Schilling, J.W., Scarborough, R.M., Lewicki, J.A., and Schenk, D.B. (1988): Atrial natriuretic peptide clearance receptor: complete sequence and functional expression of cDNA clones. J. Biol. Chem. 263, 9395-9401.

Garbers, D.L. (1988): Signal/transduction mechanisms of sea urchin spermatozoa. ISI Atlas of Science: Biochemistry 1, 120-126.

Gilman, A.G. (1987): G proteins: transducers of receptor-generated signals. Ann. Rev. Biochem. 56, 615-649.

Inagami, T. (1989): Atrial natriuretic factor. J. Biol Chem. 264, 3043-3046.

Ishido, M., Fujita, T., Shimonaka, M., Saheki, T., Ohuchi, S., Kume, T., Ishigaki, I., and Hirose, S. (1989): Inhibition of atrial natriuretic peptide-induced cyclic GMP accumulation in the bovine endothelial cells with anti-atrial natriuretic peptide receptor antiserum. J. Biol. Chem. 264, 641-645.

Kataoka, T., Broek, D., and Wigler, M. (1985): DNA sequence and characterization of the S. cerevisiae gene encoding adenylate cyclase. Cell 43, 493-505.

Koesling, D., Herz, J., Gausepohl, H., Niroomand, F., Hinsch, K.-D., Mulsch, A., Bohme, E., Schultz, G., and Frank, R. (1988): The primary structure of the 70 kDa subunit of bovine soluble guanylate cyclase. FEBS Lett. 239, 29-34.

Leitman, D.C., Andresen, J.W., Kuno, T., Kamisaki, Y., Chang, J.-K., and Murad, F. (1986): Identification of multiple binding sites for atrial natriuretic factor by affinity cross-linking in cultured endothelial cells. J. Biol. Chem. 261, 11650-11655.

Lowe, D.G., Chang, M.-S., Hellmiss, R., Chen, E., Singh, S., Garbers, D.L., and Goeddel, D.V. (1989): Human atrial natriuretic peptide receptor defines a new paradigm for second messenger signal transduction. EMBO J. 8, 1377-1384.

Maack, T., Suzuki, M., Almeida, F.A., Nossenzweig, D., Scarborough, M., McEnroe, G.A., and Lewicki, J.A. (1987): Physiological role of silent receptors of atrial natriuretic factor. Science 238, 675-678.

Nakane, M., Saheki, S., Kuno, T., Ishii, K., and Murad, F. (1988): Molecular cloning of a cDNA coding for 70 kilodalton subunit of soluble guanylate cyclase from rat lung. Biochem. Biophys. Res. Commun. 157, 1139-1147.

Shimomura, H., Dangott, L.J., and Garbers, D.L. (1986): Covalent coupling of a resact analogue to guanylate cyclase. J. Biol Chem. 261, 15778-15782.

Singh, S., Lowe, D.G., Thorpe, D.S., Rodriguez, H., Kuang, W.-J., Dangott, L.J., Chinkers, M., Goeddel, D.V., and Garbers, D.L. (1988): Membrane guanylate cyclase is a cell-surface receptor with homology to protein kinases. Nature 334, 708-712.

Thorpe, D.S., and Garbers, D.L. (1989): The membrane form of guanylate cyclase: homology with a subunit of the cytoplasmic form of the enzyme. J. Biol. Chem. 264, 6545-6549.

Hormones and Cell Regulation. N° 14, Eds J. Nunez, J.E. Dumont. Oolloque INSERM/J. Libbey Eurotext Ltd. © 1989. Vol. 198, pp. 7-13

Transmembrane signal transduction in *Dictyostelium mutans*

Peter J.M. Van Haastert

Department of Biochemistry, University of Groningen, Nijenborgh 16, 9747 AG Groningen, the Netherlands

Transmembrane signal transduction is characterized largely by the interaction between its components: ligand, receptor on the surface of cells, G-protein subunits at the inner face of the plasma membrane, and effector enzymes. The effector enzymes may vary widely depending on the organism and the ligand, and may include adenylate cyclase, guanylate cyclase, phospholipase C, and ion channels. The consequence of these interactions is the production of intracellular second messengers, such as cAMP, cGMP, inositol 1,4,5-trisphosphate [$Ins(1,4,5)P_3$], diacylglycerol, Ca^{2+}, and K^+. Besides the interaction between these proteins that generate second messengers, there also excists an extensive interaction between the second messenger systems such that one system modulates or rules another system. The main problem for the elucidation of transmembrane signal transduction is probably to understand how the flow of information proceeds through this complicated network of interacting molecules. Mutants have been shown to be very useful to unravel complex biochemical pathways. Microorganisms are most useful in this respect, since they are easy to grow, have short generation times, and have a relatively small genome which is expressed in a haploid stage.

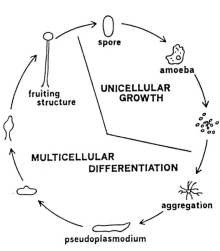

Fig. 1 The life cycle of Dictyostelium. Dictyostelium cells live in the soil as single amoebae and feed on bacteria. Exhaustion of the food source induces a developmental program: cells aggregate by means of a chemotactic reaction to a compound which is secreted by the starving cells. The aggregate may contain upto 100,000 cells, which are organized in a spatial pattern; about one third of the cell mass at the front differentiate to prestalk cells, while about two third of the cells differentiate to prespore cells. By means of morphogenetic movement and final differentiation of the cells a fruiting body is formed that is composed of spores that are embedded in a slime droplet on top of a cylinder of vacuolized dead stalk cells.

Transmembrane signal transduction has been studied extensively in the eukaryotic microorganism Dictyostelium discoideum, and appears to be very similar to signal transduction in higher eukaryotes (see Janssens and Van Haastert, 1987). Cyclic AMP is the extracellular signal in Dictyostelium, to be compared with the hormone in mammalian cells. Cyclic AMP is detected by surface receptors that have the classical seven putative transmembrane spanning domains of receptors that interact with G-proteins (Klein et al., 1988). The effector enzymes are adenylate cyclase, guanylate cyclase, and phospholipase C; the second messengers interact with target enzymes, such as protein kinases, calcium channels, and cytoskeletal components. The two main cellular functions of extracellular cAMP in Dictyostelium are chemotaxis to bring the amoeboid cells in a multicellular structure, and cell type specific gene expression to induce differentiation in this structure. Transmembrane signal transduction has been analysed in several mutants; the combination of genetic and biochemical data may provide clues on how signal transduction operates in a living cell. There are two types of mutants: mutagenized cells with the subsequent selection and characterization, and cell lines that are transformed with cloned genes such that the gene is over or underexpressed. The data are summarized in Table 1, and a model on signal transduction is presented in Fig. 2.

Mutant PsA was characterized by Brachet et al. (1979), and appears to be defective in the phosphodiesterase that is located on the surface of Dictyostelium cells. The mutant has been rescued by transformation with the phosphodiesterase gene (Podgorski et al., 1988). As a consequence of the low phosphodiesterase activity in the PsA mutant, extracellular cAMP is no longer degraded, and cells can not aggregate because they cannot detect the gradient of extracellular cAMP. However, development is normal when cells are incubated under conditions that extracellular cAMP cannot accumulate (e.g. by having a few cells in a large volume), indicating that cell surface phosphodiesterase is important to keep basal cAMP levels low, but the enzyme is not an essential component of the transmembrane signal transduction machinery.

Mutant HB3 was isolated by Barcley and Henderson (1986); the defective gene product has not been identified, but it is clear that the mutant is defective in the secretion of cAMP (Kesbeke and Van Haastert, 1988). As a consequence, the mutant has a weak capacity to aggregate and differentiate. The transduction of the cAMP signal over the plasma membrane and the induction of cellular responses is essentially unaltered in this mutant, confirming the data with the previous mutant that extracellular cAMP is the signal molecule with no other function.

Mutant stm F was characterized by Ross and Newell (1981) and is defective in the enzyme cGMP-stimulated cGMP-phosphodiesterase (Van Haastert et al., 1982). This enzyme degrades the intracellular cGMP that is formed after stimulation of the surface receptor. cGMP levels increase to very high levels in this mutant; this phenotype is accompanied with an altered chemotactic reaction and with an increased association of myosin with the triton-insoluble cytoskeleton; interestingly, the association of actin with the same cytoskeleton is not altered in mutant stm F (Liu and Newell, 1988). The activation of adenylate cyclase, guanylate cyclace and phospholipase C are not altered in mutant stm F (unpubl. observ.), suggesting that intracellular cGMP has only down-stream effects and does not influece the transmembrane sensory transduction part.

Mutant synag 7 was isolated by Frantz (1980) and addressed as N7 originally. The mutant is characterized by its defect to activate adenylate cyclase by cAMP in vivo or by GTP in vitro (Theibert and Devreotes, 1986; Van Haastert et al., 1987). The defective protein appears to be a cytosolic component that is essential for the loading of a G-protein with GTP (Snaar-Jagalska and Van Haastert, 1988), and is called GRP for Guanine nucleotide Reconstituting Protein. GRP shows some functional similarities with GAP, the GTPase activating protein of RAS (McCormick, 1989). Mutant synag 7 shows normal chemotaxis and differentiation, provided that the proper cAMP signals are given, indicating that interacellular cAMP elevations are not essential for chemotaxis and differentiation (Schaap et al., 1986; Mann and Firtel, 1989). In addition, the generation of a cGMP and Ins(1,4,5)P3 response are perfectly normal in this mutant (Schaap et al., 1986; unpubl. observ.); this demonstrates that there does not excist a feedback loop from intracellular cAMP to guanylate cyclase or phospholipase C. Mutant synag 7 belongs to a selection group that cannot aggregate by itself, but will synergize with wild-type cells (mutant PsA and HB3 also belong to this group). Such mutants are supposed to be defective in the generation of cAMP

TABLE 1. DICTYOSTELIUM SIGNAL TRANSDUCTION MUTANTS

Development of the mutants was investigated by plating the cells on hydrophobic agar and recording the formation of aggregates (agg). Cells were also analysed for the formation of cell type specific mRNAs (see Schaap et al, 1986; Mann and Firtel, 1989); these aspects of differentiation were investigated in cells in suspension in the absence and presense of cAMP pulses, respectively (diff). Responses were investigated with standard assays (see Janssens and Van Haastert, 1987): chemotaxis was measured with the small population assay; the cAMP response (CA) was measured with thew 2'deoxy cAMP method; the cGMP response (cG) was determined as described; finally, the Ins(1,4,5)P3 response was measured by HPLC of [³H]inositol-labelled cells (Van Haastert et al., 1989) or by isotope dillution assay (Van Haastert, 1989).

Mutant/protein	development		responses				remarks
	agg	diff	chem	cA	cG	ip3	
PsA/cA-PDE	−	−,+	+	+	+	+	i)
HB3/?	+	+,+	+	+	+	?	ii)
synag7/GRP	−	−,+	+	−	+	+	iii)
stmF/cG-PDE	+	+,+	++	+	++	?	
fgdA/Gα-2	−	−,−	−	−	−	−	iv)
O.E. cA-PDE	−	−,+	?	?	?	?	
A.S. cA-Rec	−	−,−	−	−	−	?	

The mutants are described in the text; O.E. and A.S. denote overexpression and antisense, respectively. The symbols denote (−), absent; (±) response strongly reduced, but not completely absent; (+), response as in wild-type; (++), response stronger than in wild-type; (?), not determined. Remarks: i) The phenotype of this mutant is restored by addition of the phosphodiesterase protein to the suspension or by transformastion of the mutant with the phosphodiesterase gene. ii) The secretion of cAMP is the main defect in this mutant. iii) GRP is a solluble protein that is essential for the loading and/or activation of a G protein with GTP. iv) Ins(1,4,5)P3 restores the acvtivation of adenylate cyclase in permeabilyzed cells, provided that the cAMP receptor is stimulated simultaneously. See text for references where appropriate.

signals, but not in the generation of second messengers that are required for chemotaxis and differentiation. Thus by isolating the synag mutants all components of the adenylate activation pathway may be found (work in progress by Puppilo, Coukell and Devreotes)

Mutants of the complementation group fgd A are probably the most interesting for for the present discussion and were isolated by Coukell et al. (1983). These mutants have normal surface cAMP receptors, but cAMP is unable to induce any cellular response with the exception of receptor phosphorylation and down regulation; furthermore, GTP inhibition of cAMP-binding and cAMP stimulation of GTPτS-binding and GTPase are strongly reduced in mutant membranes (Kesbeke et al., 1988). The mutant lacks a G-protein α-subunit as determined by Western blots with a polyclonal serum prepared against the most conserved domains of Gα (Snaar-Jagalska et al., 1988). Recently it was demonstrated that one allele of the fgd A complementation group has a 2.2 Kb deletion in one of the two genes that code for Gα-subunits (Gα-2, Pupillo et al., 1989; Kumagai et al., 1989). In this mutant GTP-stimulation of adenylate cyclase is normal, but GTP-stimulation of phospholipase C is defective, suggesting that Gα-2 couples to the inositol pathway. Interestingly, in permeabilized cells of this mutant, adenylate cyclase can be activated by the receptor, but only when Ins(1,4,5)P₃ is added simultaneously with cAMP, suggesting that in vivo the activation of the adenylate cyclase pathway requires the co-activation of the inositol pathway (Snaar-Jagalska et al., 1988).

The advent of modern molecular biology has helped to construct cell lines with an altered expression of specific genes; reduced expression has been demonstrated for several genes using antisense mRNA inactivation, or gene disruption or replacement by homologous recombination (DeLozanne and Spudich, 1987; Knecht and Loomis, 1987; Witke et al., 1987). Also overexpression of certain genes may lead to a clear phenotype. Overproduction of phosphodiesterase leads to abbarrant cell aggregation and differentiation (Podgorski et al., 1988). Inactivation of the cAMP receptor by antisence mRNA inactivation results in the expected phenotype: all signal transduction ceases. On the other hand, overexpression of the receptor leads only to a subtle phenotype (Klein et al., 1988). Cell lines with altered expression of G proteins have not yet been investigated extensively, but preliminary experiments predict strong effects (Kumagai et al., 1989). Most transformants have been generated down-stream of the transmembrane transduction pathway, in genes that code for components of the cytoskeleton (myosin heavy chain, [alpha]actinin, gelsollin). Inactivation of these genes has no decearnable effect on transmembrane signal transduction, and only relatively subtle effects on locomotion and chemotaxis (Witke et al., 1987; Noegel, pers. commun.).

Besides genetic data, there is also a wealth of biochemical data on transmembrane signal transduction in Dictyostelium (see Janssens and Van Haastert, 1987; Van Haastert, 1989). Kinetic studies show at least two sub-types of surface cAMP receptors that are supposed to couple to respectively the adenylate cyclase pathway and the guanylate cyclase/phospholipase C pathway. It is not yet clear whether these different forms of the receptor are also coded by different genes. The activation of adenylate cyclase is certainly very complex in Dictyostelium, more complex than the β-adrenergic system, but perhaps similar to the situation in leukocytes. Biochemical data suggest the presense of Gs and Gi-like activities, but their genes have not been cloned yet. Mutant synag 7 has demonstrated the requirement of an additional protein, GRP that is needed to activate the adenylate cyclase-coupled G-protein. In addition, some component of the inositol pathway is essential to activate adenylate cyclase; this component could be

Ins(1,4,5)P₃, a metabolite of Ins(1,4,5)P₃, or Ca²⁺. Studies with mutant
<u>fgd</u> A have also shown that phospholipase C and guanylate cyclase are
activated through a common step, Gα-2. It was proposed that guanylate
cyclase is activated by Ins(1,4,5)P₃-liberated Ca²⁺ (Europe-Finner et al.
1987); this is contradicted by the recent finding that submicromolar Ca²⁺
concentrations completely inactivate guanylate cyclase activity in vitro
(Janssens et al., 1989) and in permeabilized cells (unpubl. obser.). The
present data suggest that the activation of the inositol cycle is the most
important sensory transduction pathway; defects in the G-protein that
presumably activates this pathway stops all sensory transduction in
Dictyostelium. Although investigations of this pathway are not yet
complete, several peculiarities have already been demonstrated, such as the
absense of an Ins(1,4,5)P₃ 3-kinase, and an additional phosphatase that
degrade Ins(1,4,5)P₃ specifically at the one position. Ins(1,4,5)P₃
releases Ca²⁺ from internal stores; among others, Ca²⁺ participates in the
association of actin with the cytoskeleton (Europe-Finner and Newell,
1987). On the other hand, cGMP is involved in the association of myosin
with this cytoskeleton (Liu and Newell, 1988).

The combination of biochemical and genetic data suggest that cAMP signal
transduction may be composed of two parts: the adenylate cyclase pathway
that generates the extracellular cAMP signal, but has no intracellular
function known presently. The second part is the guanylate cyclase/inositol
pathway that appears to regulate chemotaxis and differentiation; this
pathway also regulates the adenylate cyclase pathway.

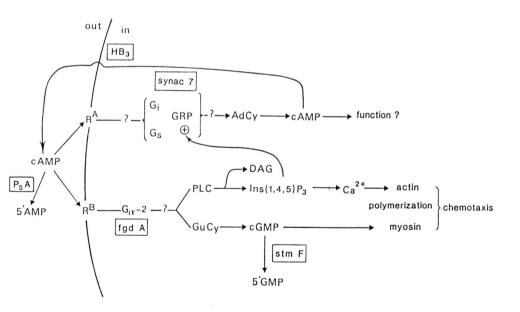

Fig. 2. Model of sensory transduction pathways in Dictyostelium. The
localization of the defects in the mutants is indicated by boxes. The
abbreviations are: R, receptor;G, G-protein; GRP, a protein defective in
mutant synac 7; AdCy, adenylate cyclase; GuCy, guanylate cyclase, PLC,
phospholipase C; DAG, diacylglycerol.

It is expected that with the present and coming cloning of signal transduction components more cell lines will become availlable in which these components are over- and underexpressed. It should be mentioned however that the classical mutants remain valuable, mainly because they have the potention to ellucidate components that are unknown presently; e.g. the protein that is defective in mutant synag 7 would not have been easily detected and characterized without this mutant. Mutants with defects down-stream of the second messengers are also badly needed. We have recently characterized a mutant that is essentially normal in all aspects of transmembrane signal transduction, but is defective in cAMP induced gene expression. These mutants become even more valuable if they can be rescued by complementation with a wild-type genomic library. Indeed, it is the combination of powerful biochemical and genetic methods that allows Dictyostelium to be an organism in which the intricate nettwork of sensory transduction pathways can be understood.

ACKNOWLEDGEMENTS

I thank Fanja Kesbeke, Ewa Snaar, and Anthony Bominaar for helpful suggestions. This work was supported by a grant of the C. and C. Huygens Fund which is subsidized by the Netherlands Organization of Scientific Research.

REFERENCES

Barcley, S.L., and Henderson, E.J. (1986). Altered cAMP receptor activity and morphogenesis in a chemosensory mutant of Dictyostelium discoideum. Differentiation 33, 111-120.

Coukell, M.B., Lappano, S., and Cameron, A.M. (1983). Isolation and characterization of cAMP unresponsive (frigid) aggregation-deficient mutants of Dictyostelium discoideum. Dev. Genet. 3, 283-297.

De Lozanne, A., and Spudich, J. (1987). Disruption of the Dictyostelium myosin heavy chain gene by homologous recombination. Science 236, 1086-1091.

Europe-Finner, G.N., and Newell, P.C. (1985). Inositol 1,4,5-trisphosphate induces cyclic GMP formation in Dictyostelium discoideum. Biochem. Biophys. Res. Commun. 130, 1115-1122.

Europe-Finner, G.N., and Newell, P.C. (1986). Inositol 1,4,5-trisphosphate and calcium induce actin polymerization in Dictyostelium discoideum. J. Cell Sci. 82, 41-51.

Frantz, C.E. (1980). Phenotype analysis of aggregation mutants of Dictyostelium discoideum. PhD thesis, University of Chicago.

Janssens, P.M.W., De Jong, C.C.C., Vink, A.A., and Van Haastert, P.J.M. (1989) The regulation of a magnesium-dependent guanylate cyclase in Dictyostelium membranes. J. Biol. Chem., in press.

Janssens, P.M.W., and Van Haastert, P.J.M. (1987). Molecular basis of transmembrane signal transduction in Dictyostelium discoideum. Microbiol. Rev. 51, 396-418.

Kesbeke, F., Snaar-Jagalska, B.E., and Van Haastert, P.J.M. (1988). Signal transduction in Dictyostelium fgdA mutants with a defective interaction between surface cAMP receptor and a GTP binding regulatory protein. J. Cell Biol. 107, 521-528.

Kesbeke, F., and Van Haastert, P.J.M. (1988). Reduced cAMP secretion in Dictyostelium discoideum mutant HB3. Dev. Biol. 130, 464-470.

Klein, P., Sun, T.J., Saxe, C.L., Kimmel, A.R., and Devreotes, P.N. (1989). A chemoattractant receptor controls development in Dictyostelium discoideum. Science, 241, 1467-1472.

Knecht, D.A., and Loomis, W.A. (1987). Antisense RNA inactivation of myosin heavy chain gene expression in Dictyostelium discoideum. Science 236, 1081-1086.

Kumagai, A., Pupillo, M., Gunderson, R., Mike-Lye, R., Devreotes, P.N., and Firtel, R.A. (1989). Regulation and function of G_α protein subunits in Dictyostelium. Cell, 57, 265-275.

Liu, G., and Newell, P.C. (1988). Evidence that cGMP regulates myosin interaction with the cytoskeleton during chemotaxis of Dictyostelium. J. Cell Sci. 90, 123-129.

McCormick, F. (1989). ras GTPase activating protein: signal transmitter and signal terminator. Cell 56, 5-8.

Mann, S.K.O., and Firtel, R.A. (1989) Two-phase regulatory pathway controls cAMP-mediated expression of early genes in Dictyostelium. Proc. Natl. Acad. Sci. USA. 86, 1924-1928.

Podgorski, G.J., Faure, M., Franke, J., and Kessin, R.H. (1988). The cyclic nucleotide phosphodiesterase of Dictyostelium discoideum: The structure of ther gene and its regulation and role in development. Dev. Gen. 9, 267-278.

Pupillo, M., Kumagai, A., Pitt, G., Firtel, R.A., and Devreotes, P.N. (1989). Multiple αsubunits of G proteins in Dictyostelium. Proc. Natl. Acad. Sci. USA, in press.

Ross, F.M., and Newell, P.C. (1981). Streamers: chemotactic mutants of Dictyostelium with altered cyclic GMP metabolism. J. Gen. Microbiol. 127, 339-343.

Schaap, P., Van Lookeren Campagne, M.M., Van Driel, R., Spek, W., Van Haastert, P.J.M., and Pinas, J.E. (1986). Postaggregative differentiation induction by cyclic AMP in Dictyostelium: Intracellullar transduction pathway and requirement for additional stimuli. Dev. Biol. 118, 52-63.

Small, N.V., Europe-Finner, G.N., and Newell, P.C. (1986). Calcium induces cyclic GMP formation in Dictyostelium. FEBS Lett. 203, 11-14.

Snaar-Jagalska, B.E., Kesbeke, F., and Van Haastert, P.J.M. (1988). G proteins in the signal transduction pathways of Dictyostelium discoideum. Dev. Genet. 9, 215-226.

Snaar-Jagalka, B.E., Kesbeke, F. Pupillo, M., and Van Haastert, P.J.M. (1988). Immunological detection of G protein α subunits in Dictyostelium discoideum. Biochem. Biophys. Res. Commun. 156, 757-761

Snaar-Jagalska, B.E., and Van Haastert, P.J.M. (1988) Dictyostelium discoideum mutant synag 7 with altered G-protein adenylate cyclase interaction. J. Cell Sci. 91, 287-294.

Theibert, A., and Devreotes, P.N. (1986). Surface receptor mediated activation of adenylate cyclase in Dictyostelium is regulated by guanylnucleotides; mutant characterization, and in vitro mutant reconstitution. J. Biol. Chem. 261, 15121-15125.

Van Haastert, P.J.M. (1989) Sensory transduction pathways in Dictyostelium. Adv. Cycl. Nucl. Res, in press.

Van Haastert, P.J.M., Snaar-Jagalska, B.E., and Janssens, P.M.W. (1987). The regulation of adenylate cyclase by guanine nucleotides in Dictyostelium discoideum membranes. Eur. J. Biochem. 162, 251-258.

Van Haastert, P.J.M., Van Lookeren Campagne, M.M., and Ross, F.M. (1982). Altered cGMP-phosphodiesterase activity in chemotactic mutants of Dictyostelium discoideum. FEBS Lett. 147, 149-152.

Witke, W., Nellen, W., and Noegel, A. (1987). Homologous recombination in the Dictyostelium α-actinin gene leads to an altered mRNA and lack of the protein. EMBO J. 6, 4143-4148.

Hormones and Cell Regulation. N° 14, Eds J. Nunez, J.E. Dumont. Colloque INSERM/J. Libbey Eurotext Ltd. © 1989. Vol. 198, pp. 15-20

Ca++ requirement of MSH-receptor function : an unusual example among G-protein-associated peptide hormone receptors

Yoram Salomon

Department of Hormone Research, The Weizmann Institute of Science, Rehovot 76100, Israel

Melanotropins are being traditionally associated with the control of pigmentation in vertebrates. Yet, there are three homologous melanocyte-stimulating hormone (MSH) peptides (αMSH, βMSH and γMSH), the differential function of which is not well-defined. In addition, adrenocorticotropic hormone (ACTH), another bioactive derivative of proopiomelanocortin (POMC) is conventionally associated with the control of adrenal steroidogenesis. This peptide contains the entire amino acid sequence of αMSH and is able to stimulate melanogenesis under certain circumstances.

The synthesis and processing of POMC have been described in recent years, not only in the pituitary, its major site of synthesis, but also in the central nervous system and in peripheral tissues (Smith & Funder, 1988). Furthermore, it has become apparent that the melanocortin peptides (α-, β-, γMSH and ACTH) are involved in the control of various biological processes that are not associated with their classical endocrine role as hormones of the pituitary. These peptides induce a host of behavioral effects when tested in experimental animals and humans (De Wied & Ferrari, 1986; De Wied & Jolles, 1982), facilitate nerve regeneration (Bijlsma *et al.*, 1983a; Dekker *et al.*, 1987) and recovery of motor performance in rats following crush denervation (Saint-Come *et al.*, 1982; Strand *et al.*, 1981; Bijlsma *et al.*, 1981; Bijlsma *et al.*, 1983b; Bijlsma *et al.*, 1984), cause long-lasting potentiation of transmitter release in motor nerve terminals (Johnston *et al.*, 1983), and increase the miniature end-plate potential in the neuromuscular junction (Strand *et al.*, 1981). MSH and ACTH have recently been shown also to stimulate lacrimal secretion in the rat (Jahn et al., 1982).

In order to understand the molecular basis of the function of melanocortins and to elucidate their role in such diverse processes, it is necessary to study the receptor entities that mediate their function.

MSH regulates melanocytic functions such as melanin synthesis and cell growth, by controlling cellular cyclic AMP levels (Eberle, 1988). We used the M2R mouse melanoma cell line (Gerst *et al.*, 1986) as the subject of our studies on this receptor in pigment cells.

In a competition binding study using [125I]iodo porcine βMSH, we found that βMSH, αMSH and ACTH$_{1-24}$ are equipotent in binding to the cellular M2R cell receptor with a Kd of ~20 nM (Gerst et al., 1986). Elevation of cAMP levels by βMSH in intact cells, as well as activity of adenylate cyclase (AC) in a cell membrane preparation, were saturable, dose-dependent and correlated well with the binding affinity of the receptor for the hormone. Receptor density was 75,000/cell or 1 pmol/mg membrane protein. Receptor affinity for βMSH in membrane preparations was reduced substantially by GTP or its analogues (Gerst et al., 1987). This finding indicated that, in the pathway leading to AC activation, the molecular interactions distal to the MSH-receptor, i.e., G-protein activation, are probably similar to other peptide hormone receptors (Rodbell, 1980). Of special interest was the unusual behavior of the MSH-receptor when ambient calcium concentrations were manipulated (Gerst et al., 1987). When we reduced free Ca^{++} concentrations in the medium to below 15 nM using calculated EGTA concentrations, MSH no longer elevated cyclic AMP levels in intact melanocytes and at concentrations <10 nM did not activate adenylate cyclase in cell membrane preparations. Upon gradual replenishment of Ca^{++} ion concentrations to 1 mM, the responsiveness to MSH recovered in a dose-dependent manner, showing two Ca^{++}-dependency sites. Fifteen percent of the response level exhibited by the control cells recovered at 10 μM free Ca^{++} (ED$_{50}$ = 1 μM). Further elevation of free Ca^{++} concentration increased the response by another 6-7-fold to the level observed in control cells and represented the major calcium effect saturating at 0.5 mM free Ca^{++} (ED$_{50}$ = ~0.05 mM). Concurrently, under identical conditions, cyclic AMP production, in response to prostaglandin E$_1$ (PGE$_1$), was unaffected by the variation in Ca^{++} concentrations. Assuming that G-protein regulation of AC is identical for both receptor systems, we concluded that the Ca^{++}-requiring step in this regulatory pathway must be proximal to G-protein activation and suggested that MSH-receptor activity requires Ca++ (Gerst et al., 1987). It was, therefore, logical to examine whether MSH-receptor binding activity requires Ca^{++} ions. Indeed, when monitoring [125I]iodo βMSH binding under similar incubation conditions, we were surprised to find an identical Ca^{++} concentration dependence. Further analysis of this process revealed that the mechanism, whereby Ca^{++} controls MSH-receptor function, is by affinity modulation. Thus, the affinity of the receptor for MSH (Kd) increased 20-fold, from 400 nM in the absence to 20 nM in the presence of Ca^{++}. This dramatic effect of Ca^{++} was not only confined to association of the receptor with βMSH, but was also seen using the αMSH super-agonist, [Nle^{4}DPhe^7]αMSH (Salomon, Y., unpublished). Although we experimentally manipulated extracellular Ca^{++} concentrations, the location of the relevant Ca^{++} dependency sites and their distribution between the intra- and extracellular compartments have not yet been clarified. In comparison to the effect of other divalent cations on MSH binding, Ca^{++} was found to be preferable (Ca^{++} > Sr^{++} ≥ Ni ≥ Ba^{++} >> Mn^{++} > Cd^{++} > Co^{++} > Cu^{++} >> Mg^{++}), suggesting it as the likely physiological regulator of MSH-receptor activity. The effect of Ca^{++} on MSH binding was rapid and reversible. Preformed receptor-MSH complexes dissociated readily (within seconds) upon elimination of ambient Ca^{++} and reformed upon replenishment of Ca^{++}, implicating a dynamic adjustment of the extent of receptor occupancy with varying Ca^{++} concentrations. These experiments also demonstrated that the receptor-MSH complex exists in a high-affinity calcium containing state and in a low-affinity calcium-depleted state. Inter-conversion between these states required receptor-MSH complex dissociation and was not simply achieved by association/dissociation of Ca^{++} (Gerst et al., 1987).

To examine the nature of the Ca^{++}-mediating component, we investigated whether Calmodulin (CaM) or a similar Ca^{++}-binding protein may be involved in MSH-receptor activity. This was assessed by studying the effects of two classes of CaM antagonists on MSH-receptor function. It was first found that Fluphenazine selectively inhibited (ED$_{50}$ = 16 μM) the binding of MSH. Fluphenazine (100 μM) totally blocked AC stimulation by MSH, but had only a marginal effect on stimulation of the enzyme by PGE$_1$ (Gerst & Salomon, 1987). Similarly, we observed that Melittin, a bee venom-derived CaM-binding peptide (ED$_{50}$ = 2.4 μM) (Gerst & Salomon, 1987), as well as the synthetic 17-amino-acid CaM-binding peptide (M5) (ED$_{50}$ = 1 μM) comprising the C-terminus of Myosin Light Chain Kinase, both inhibited MSH-receptor functions (binding and stimulation of AC) in a selective manner (Gerst & Salomon, 1988). Their effects were non-competitive with respect to MSH concentrations, suggesting that both of these peptides do not compete for the MSH-binding domain, but rather interact elsewhere. While these results are suggestive of the possible involvement of a CaM-type component in MSH-receptor function, further experimentation is still required to elucidate the mechanism and directly identify the site responsible for the observed Ca^{++} effects.

In other experiments, we identified the MSH-receptor entity in M2R cells by photoaffinity labeling using azido[^{125}I]iodo βMSH. These experiments revealed a 44 KDa protein doublet that was specifically labeled. Covalent protein labeling was selectively inhibited by EGTA and GTPγS and dose-dependently (ED$_{50}$ = 45 μM) by unlabeled βMSH, but unaffected by VIP (Gerst et al., 1988). The strong resemblance of these results to the pharmacological profile of the receptor suggests that the photoaffinity labeled protein is the MSH-receptor. Similar conclusions were reached by Scimonelli & Eberle (1987).

As a model for MSH-receptor activity in non-melanogenic tissue, we used the rat lacrimal gland. This tissue has been reported by Jahn et al. (1982) to be stimulated by MSH and ACTH in terms of cyclic AMP production and protein secretion. Using [^{125}I]iodo[Nle^{4}DPhe^7]αMSH, we determined KD = 0.8 nM and a maximal binding capacity of ~100 fmol MSH/mg membrane protein using a 10,000-30,000 x g lacrimal membrane pellet. We found that the rat lacrimal MSH-receptor is confined to acinar cells (Salomon et al., 1989) and showed a different pharmacological profile than its melanoma counterpart. While αMSH and ACTH$_{1-24}$ competed equally well with the radioligand (ED$_{50}$ = 100 nM) and unlabeled [Nle^{4}DPhe^7]αMSH competed extremely efficiently (ED$_{50}$ = 0.5 nM), porcine βMSH was unable, at concentrations exceeding 1 μM, to compete for receptor binding. This result suggests that the MSH-receptor in this tissue probably represents a different receptor subclass. However, in spite of the implied difference in the receptor type, MSH binding was Ca^{++}-dependent (ED$_{50}$ = 0.2 mM) and was inhibited by Melittin (ED$_{50}$ = 2 μM) and the M5 peptide (ED$_{50}$ = 1 μM). These properties seem, therefore, to be common and inherent to both types of MSH-receptors.

Other reports, suggesting the need for Ca^{++} in MSH control in lower vertebrates, have been detailed earlier (Vesely & Hadley, 1971; De Graan et al., 1982). Similarly, a Ca^{++}-dependency was described for adrenocortical ACTH receptors (Lefkowitz et al., 1970). It is clearly demonstrated by us now that, in addition to the negative affinity modulation afforded from the cytoplasmic compartment by GTP via the G-protein on hormone-receptors, the positive control by Ca^{++}

in the case of the MSH-receptor apparently operates from the extra-cellular milieu.

Ca^{++} concentrations in extracellular fluids is thought to be homeo-static at 1-2 mM. Consequently, it does not seem obvious that sig-nificant variations in concentration of extracellular free Ca^{++}, that could affect melanocortin-receptor function, would exist. However, the activity of several hormone receptors has been reported to be regulated by cations found in the extracellular fluid. The binding of agonist to the catecholamine α_2 receptor (Tsai & Lefkowitz, 1978), the muscarinic cholinergic receptor (Rosenberger et al., 1980), as well as the binding of opiates (Pert & Snyder, 1974), have been reported to be inhibited by Na^+, a cation of extreme abundance in extracellular fluids. β-adreno- receptors, on the other hand, have been found to be stimulated by extracellular Na+ (Heidenreich et al., 1980). How and where can Ca^{++} then be envisaged to play a modulatory role on MSH in vivo?

We (Gerst et al., 1989) and others (Panasci et al., 1987; Eberle, 1988) have described conditions whereby receptor-MSH complexes are internalized in cultured melanocytes. This universal process reflects both receptor turnover, as well as hormone-induced down-regulation, a process that among other things enhances dissociation of the receptor-hormone complex en route to receptor reutilization and/or hormone degradation.

Before pinching off into the cytoplasmic space, free Ca^{++} ion con-centrations in the growing endosome are those found in the extracel-lular space. However, Ca^{++} concentrations in the newly formed endocytic vesicle rapidly drop and approach intracellular free Ca^{++} levels (submicromolar range) as a result of rapid equilibration bet-ween the endocytic inner compartment and the cell cytoplasm. It is, therefore, anticipated that, under such circumstances, conditions may be created that would specifically enhance rapid melanocortin disso-ciation within the endosome. Most peptides, including MSH, as well as glycoprotein hormones (Amir & Salomon, 1980), are thought to disso-ciate due to acidification under similar circumstances. The anticipa-ted rapid drop in Ca^{++} concentrations in the endocytic environment can, therefore, be suggested to selectively terminate melanocortin stimulation. Such a situation may be of importance primarily in relation to the yet unexplained involvement of these peptides in the neuronal activity, notably their role as neurotransmitters or neuromodulators.

With regard to the last point, it is of interest to note that non-homogenous Ca^{++} ion concentrations within the synaptic space are thought to be associated with the regulation of synaptic activity (Ginsburg & Rahamimoff, 1983). Consequently, conditions envisaged as influencing melanocortin activity may temporarily exist within this compartment and modulate peptide activity, thus affecting transmitter release (Johnston et al., 1983). The possibility, that the described Ca^{++} dependency of the MSH-receptor, as seen by us in vitro, reflects a process controlled by other regulators in vivo, cannot be excluded at this point. Yet, we believe that this feature of the MSH-receptor represents a unique property among G-protein-associated peptide hor-mone receptors, the full physiological significance of which has yet to be fully explored.

ACKNOWLEDGEMENT

I wish to acknowledge the devoted secretarial assistance of Rachel Benjamin, and the contributions of J.E. Gerst, J. Schmidt-Sole, N.B. Garty, H. Leiba and M. Tosky. This work was supported by a grant from the Hermann and Lilly Schilling Foundation for Medical Research, F.R.G.

REFERENCES

Amir, Y. & Salomon, Y. (1980): Studies on the receptor for luteinizing hormone in a purified plasma membrane preparation from rat ovary. *Endocrinology* 106, 1166-1172.

Bijlsma, W.A., van Asselt, E., Veldman, H., Jennekens, F.G.I., Schotman, P. & Gispen, W.H. (1983a): Ultrastructural study of effect of ACTH(4-10) on nerve regeneration; axons become larger in number and smaller in diameter. *Acta Neuropathol.* 62, 24-30.

Bijlsma, W.A., Jennekens, F.G.I., Schotman, P. & Gispen, W.H. (1981): Effects of corticotropin (ACTH) on recovery of sensorimotor function in the rat: structure-activity study. *Eur. J. Pharmacol.* 76, 73-79.

Bijlsma, W.A., Jennekens, F.G.I., Schotman, P. & Gispen, W.H. (1983b): Stimulation by ACTH(4-10) of nerve fibre regeneration following sciatic nerve crush. *Muscle Nerve* 6, 104-112.

Bijlsma, W.A., Jennekens, F.G.I., Schotman, P. & Gispen, W.H. (1984): Neurotrophic factors and regeneration in the peripheral nervous system. *Psychoneuroendocrinology* 9, 199-215.

De Graan, P.N.E., Eberle, A.N. & Van de Veerdonk, F.C.G. (1982a): Calcium requirement for αMSH action on tail fin melanophores of *Xenopus* tadpoles. *Mol. Cell. Endocr.* 26, 327-329.

Dekker, A., Gispen, W.H. & De Wied, D. (1987): Axonal regeneration, growth factors and neuropeptides. *Life Sci.* 41, 1667-1678.

De Wied, D. & Ferrari, W. (Eds.) (1986): Central Actions of ACTH and Related Peptides. Symposia in Neuroscience, Vol. 4, Springer-Verlag.

De Wied, D. & Jolles, J. (1982): Neuropeptides derived from proopiomelanocortin: behavioral, physiological, and neurochemical effects. *Physiol. Rev.* 62, 976-1059.

Eberle, A.N. (Ed.) (1988): The Melanotropins: Chemistry, Physiology and Mechanisms of Action. Basel: Karger.

Gerst, J.E., Benezra, M., Schimmer, A. & Salomon, Y. (1989): Phorbol ester impairs melanotropin receptor function and stimulates growth of cultured M2R melanoma cells. *Eur. J. Pharmacol.* 172, 29-39.

Gerst, J.E. & Salomon, Y. (1987): Inhibition by melittin and fluphenazine of melanotropin receptor function and adenylate cyclase in M2R melanoma cell membranes. *Endocrinology* 121, 1766-1772.

Gerst, J.E. & Salomon, Y. (1988): A synthetic analog of the calmodulin binding domain of myosin light chain kinase inhibits melanotropin receptor function. *J. Biol. Chem.* 263, 7073-7078.

Gerst, J.E., Sole, J., Hazum, E. & Salomon, Y. (1988): Identification and characterization of melanotropin binding proteins from M2R melanoma cells by covalent photoaffinity labeling. *Endocrinology* 123, 1792-1797.

Gerst, J., Sole, J., Mather, J.P. & Salomon, Y. (1986): Regulation of adenylate cyclase by β-melanotropin in the M2R melanoma cell line. *Mol. Cell. Endocrinol.* 46, 137-147.

Gerst, J., Sole, J. & Salomon, Y. (1987): Dual regulation of β-MSH receptor function and adenylate cyclase by calcium and guanosine nucleotides in the M2R melanoma cell line. *Molec. Pharmacol.* 31, 81-88.

Ginsburg, S. & Rahamimoff, R. (1983): Is extracellular calcium buffering involved in regulation of transmitter release at the neuromuscular junction? *Nature* 306, 62-64.

Heidenreich, K.A., Weiland, G.A. & Molinoff, P.B. (1980): Characterization of radiolabeled agonist binding to β-adrenergic receptors in mammalian tissues. *J. Cyclic Nucl. Res.* 6, 217-230.

Jahn, R., Padel, U., Porsch, P.H. & Söling, H.D. (1982): Adrenocorticotropic hormone and α-melanocyte-stimulating hormon induce secretion and protein phosphorylation in the rat lacrimal gland by activation of a cAMP-dependent pathway. *Eur. J. Biochem.* 126, 623-629.

Johnston, M.F., Kravitz, E.A., Meiri, H. & Rahamimoff, R. (1983): Adrenocorticotropic hormone causes long-lasting potentiation of transmitter release from frog motor nerve terminals. *Science* 220, 1071-1072.

Lefkowitz, R.J., Roth, J. & Pastan, I. (1970): Effects of calcium on ACTH stimulation of the adrenal: separation of hormone binding from adenyl cyclase stimulation. *Nature* (London) 228, 864-866.

Panasci, L.C., McQuillan, A. & Kaufman, M. (1987): Biological activity, binding, and metabolic fate of Ac-Nle4,D-Phe7]α-MSH(4-11)MH2 with the F1 variant of B16 melanoma cells. *J. Cell Physiol.* 132, 97-103.

Pert, C. & Snyder, S. (1974): Opiate receptor binding of agonists and antagonists affected differentially by sodium. *Mol. Pharmacol.* 10, 868-879.

Rodbell, M. (1980): The role of hormone receptors and GTP-regulatory proteins in membrane transduction. *Nature* (London) 284, 17-22.

Rosenberger, L.B., Yamamura, H.I. & Roeske, W.R. (1980): Cardiac muscarinic cholinergic receptor binding is regulated by Na^+ and guanyl nucleotides. *J. Biol. Chem.* 255, 820-823.

Saint-Come, C., Acker, G.R. & Strand, F.L. (1982): Peptide influences on the development and regeneration of motor performance. *Peptides* 3, 439-449.

Salomon, Y., Leiba, H. & Garty, N.B. (1989) The MSH-receptor in the rat lacrimal gland: location and pharmacology. In *Proceedings of the Endocrine Society Meeting*, 1989, Abst.

Scimonelli, T. & Eberle, A.N. (1987): Photoaffinity labeling of melanoma cell MSH-receptors. *FEBS Lett.* 226, 134-138.

Smith, A.I. &'Funder, J.W. (1988): Proopiomelanocortin processing in the pituitary, central nervous system, and peripheral tissues. *Endocr. Rev.* 9, 159-179.

Strand, F.L., Kung, T.T. & Saint-Come, C. (1981) Regenerative ability of spinal motor systems as influences by ACTH/MSH peptides. In *Functional Recovery From Brain Damage*, ed. M.W. Van Hof & G. Mohn, pp. 369-409. North Holland: Elsevier.

Tsai, B.S. & Lefkowitz, R.J. (1978): Agonist-specific effects of monovalent and divalent cations on adenylate cyclase-coupled alpha adrenergic receptors in rabbit platelet. *Mol. Pharmacol.* 14, 540-548.

Vesely, D.L. & Hadley, M.E. (1971): Calcium requirement for melanophore-stimulating hormone action on melanophores. *Science* 173, 923-925.

Hormones and Cell Regulation. N° 14, Eds J. Nunez, J.E. Dumont. Colloque INSERM/J. Libbey Eurotext Ltd. © 1989. Vol. 198, pp. 21-26

Irreversible V2 vasopressin receptor activation : effect on down-regulation of the cAMP mediated cellular response

Falk Fahrenholz, Heike Luzius and David A. Jans

Max-Planck-Institut für Biophysik, Kennedy Allee 70, D-6000 Frankfurt am Main, FRG

Exposure of cells to hormones can lead to a diminished response despite the continued presence of stimulus. This down-regulation of a cellular response has been referred to as desensitization or hormone-induced refractoriness.

One of the first steps in desensitization of adenylate cyclase-linked receptors may involve receptor modifications by phosphorylation. Alterations of guanine nucleotide regulatory (G) proteins or the adenylate cyclase may be the site of additional functionally significant changes; the nature of such alterations, however, is at present unknown (review by Benovic et al, 1988). Such modifications of the components of the adenylate cyclase system could result in desensitization by either lowering the receptor affinity for the stimulating hormone or by a functional uncoupling of receptor, G proteins and adenylate cyclase.

Another specific mechanism for regulating hormone responsiveness represents the "down-regulation" of receptors: following more prolonged agonist stimulation, the number of plasma membrane hormone-receptor complexes is decreased by their internalization followed by the lysosomal dissociation of ligand and receptor.

Subsequent to these regulatory steps at the level of the signal transducing system, a complex series of intracellular events occurs which results in a return to the basal level of cellular response. Those down-regulatory cAMP mediated events include the stimulation of phosphodiesterase (Schwartz and Passoneau, 1974) and the removal of the free, active catalytic subunit of the cAMP-dependent protein kinase (Hemmings, 1986) possibly by a specific proteolytic mechanism.

In the mammalian kidney the antidiuretic hormone vasopressin increases water permeability of the collceting duct (CD) and enhances salt reabsorption in the thick ascending limb (TAL) of Henle'loop of the rat kidney. These responses are mediated by adenylate cyclase coupled V2 receptors. The evidence to date concerning the V2 receptor regulation indicates that desensitization occurs in the CD (Kirk, 1988) and the TAL (Elalouf, 1988). It has been ascribed to either receptor cyclase uncoupling (Rajerison et al, 1974), or to receptor affinity transition (Roy et al 1981), or to receptor internalization (Lester et al, 1985; Kirk, 1988).

We examined the process of down-regulation the cellular response following vasopressin stimulation in the LLC-PK1 cell line (Hull et al, 1976). This cell line affords an attractive possibility for such studies in that besides vasopressin the polypeptide hormone calcitonin elevates intracellular cAMP levels (Dayer et al 1981). We examined whether the irreversible binding of a photoactivatable vasopressin agonist to the V2 receptor bypasses the processes of down-regulation, thereby leading to a prolonged cAMP mediated celluar response. For this purpose we used the photoactivatable analogue of vasopressin 1-(3-mercapto) propionic acid, 8-(N6-4-azido-phenylamidino)lysine vasopressin (apa-LVP), which, without photoactivation, has an affinity for the renal V2 vasopressin receptor (Kd = 1.8 nM) almost identical to that of Arg-vasopressin (Kd = 1.1 nM) (Fahrenholz et al, 1985) and exhibits a high <u>in vivo</u> antidiuretic activity (Fahrenholz et al, 1986).

LONG TERM STIMULATION OF cAMP PRODUCTION

Cells were incubated for various times with or without hormone or apa-LVP, with or without photoactivation, the final 30 min in the presence or absence of the phosphodiesterase (PDE) inhibitor IBMX (0.5 mM). The PDE inhibitor IBMX can be used to detect continued adenylate cyclase activity subsequent to agonist stimulation, which can then be measured through activation of the cAMP-dependent protein kinase (cAMP-PK) by cAMP. A greater extent or activation of cAMP-PK (as expressed by the cAMP-PK activity ratio) in the presence than in the absence of IBMX, indicates continued production of cAMP by adenylate cyclase at the time of measurement (Lamp et al, 1981; Jans et al, 1987).

The results at various incubation times are shown in Fig. 1. 30 min treatment of the cells with apa-LVP with or without photoactivation in the presence of IBMX results in near maximal activation of cAMP-PK (activity ratios of 0.72 and 0.63

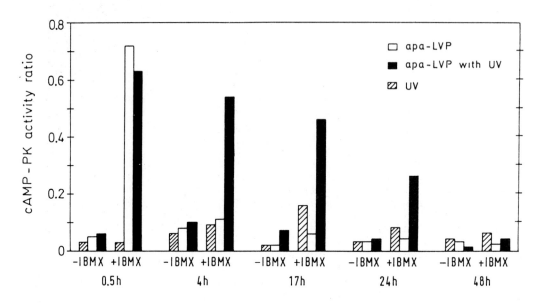

Fig. 1 Long term stimulation of cAMP production in LLC-PK1 cells treated with apa-LVP followed by photoactivation. Cells were treated and cAMP-PK activity ratio measured as described (Jans et al, 1987). ▨ Cells treated with photoactivation alone; ☐ Cells treated with apa-LVP (no photoactivation); ■ Cells treated with apa-LVP followed by photoactivation. Results represent the means for 3 separate experiments of duplicate determinations.

respectively). 4 h after treatment with apa-LVP without photoactivation, the response is already down-regulated to nearly basal levels (activity ratio 0.11). Without photoactivation, the vasopressin analogue-elicited responses were identical to those induced by vasopressin (Jans et al, 1987), in that cAMP synthesis returned to the basal unstimulated level about 4 h after hormonal treatment. Cells subjected to ultraviolet irradiation subsequent to the addition of the analogue, however, exhibited prolonged stimulation of adenylate cyclase activity. Even 24 h after the addition of apa-LVP followed by photoactivation, the cAMP-PK activity ratio was markedly higher in the presence (0.29) than in the absence (0.05) of IBMX. The same experiment was performed with the vasopressin receptor negative LLC-PK1 mutant cell line M18 (Jans et al, 1986). Ultraviolet irradiation of apa-LVP treated M18 cells induced no stimulation of cAMP production. These results implied clearly that the mediator of the persistent stimulation in LLC-PK1 cells was the V2-receptor, since M18 cells, lacking the receptor, showed no such response.

PROLONGED PRODUCTION OF PLASMINOGEN ACTIVATOR AFTER REMOVAL OF FREE LIGAND

One consequence of elevation of intracellular cAMP concentration subsequent to agonist addition is the induction of production of the urokinase-type plasminogen activator (uPA) which is extracelluarly secreted (Nagamine et al, 1983; Jans et al, 1986). LLC-PK1 were treated for 1 min with 1 nM apa-LVP or AVP, with or without subsequent photoactivation, and then washed to remove hormone, prior to incubation in serum-free medium for the periods 0-24 h or 24-48 h after treatment.

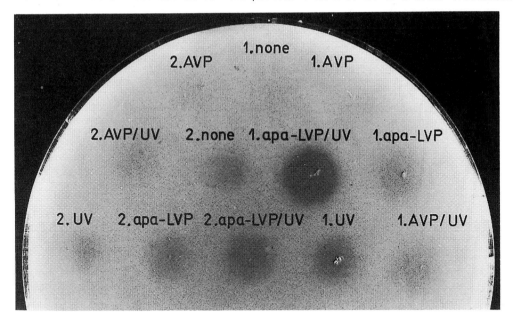

Fig. 2 uPA production by LLC-PK1 cells treated with AVP or the photoactivatable vasopressin analogue apa-LVP, with or without photoactivation. Cell monolayers were incubated with or without hormone for 1 min, with or without subsequent photoactivation, washed, and then incubated for 24 h in serum-free medium, (indicated with 1) or for 24 h in serum-containing medium, prior to washing, and incubation for a further 24 h with serum-free medium (i.e., for the period 24-48 h, indicated with 2). Medium was collected and 5 µl spotted onto a plasminogen-containing casein agar, whereby uPA activity in the medium is visible as a zone of lysis in the agar (eg.1. apa-LVP/UV).

The medium was then assayed for uPA activity by spotting onto a casein-plasminogen agar (Fig. 2). Significant uPA activity (zones of proteolytic lysis of casein in the agar) could only be detected in 0-24 h medium from cells treated with apa-LVP followed by photoactivation (Fig. 2). For the comparable time period, cells treated with apa-LVP or AVP without photoactivation, cells treated with photoactivation alone, or cells treated with AVP and photoactivation, all showed uPA production essentially comparable to control cells. Medium for the 24-48 h time period showed no detectable uPA activity (Fig. 2) above that for untreated cells. These results paralleled those for cAMP-PK activation in that only cells treated with the photoactivatable analogue and photoactivation were stimulated to a marked extent, and that down-regulation appeared to have occured after about 24 h. The results were also consistent with the idea that photoactivation of the apa-LVP analogue results in covalent binding to the receptor, since stimulation of uPA production by photoactivated apa-LVP could be demonstrated even when the ligand was removed from the medium subsequent to photoactivation.

PERISTENT STIMULATION OF ADENYLATE CYCLASE IS CYTOTOXIC TO LLC-PK1 CELLS

Prolonged elevation of intracellular cAMP levels, effected by treatment with forskolin, IBMX or cAMP analogues has a cytotoxic effect on LLC-PK1 cells (Jans and Hemmings, 1986). The photoactivated apa-LVP analogue can be shown to have similar effects (Jans et al, 1987). The LLC-PK1 and vasopressin receptor negative mutant M18 cell lines were treated with or without apa-LVP, with or without subsequent photoactivation, and cell counts performed for up to 10 days. AVP and apa-LVP without photoactivation have no effect on the growth of LLC-PK1 or M18 cells, growth resembling that for untreated cells in all respect (Jans et al, 1987). LLC-PK1 cells treated with apa-LVP and photoactivation, however, show a strong inhibition of growth, cell numbers being only 22 % those of the photoactivated control. Consistent with its lack of vasopressin binding, the M18 mutant shows no such effect, cells treated with apa-LVP and photoactivation resembling those treated with photoactivation alone, in all respects. A LLC-PK1 cell mutant in cAMP-PK was resistant to growth inhibition by the activated vasopressin analogue (Jans et al 1987) implying that the growth inhibitory effects of the prolonged stimulation of adenylate cyclase are mediated by cAMP-PK.

OTHER EXAMPLES OF LIGAND-INDUCED BYPASS OF DOWN-REGULATION

The analogue apa-LVP and similar analogues containing a photoreactive azido group either in position 3 or 8 of the vasopressin amino acid sequence, have also been shown to induce a prolonged hydro-osmotic response in the toad urinary bladder after photoactivation (Fahrenholz et al, 1983 and 1986; Eggena et al, 1983) as the result of covalent linkage to the receptor (Eggena et al, 1984).
Salmon calcitonin induces an analogous long term stimulation in both LLC-PK1 (Jans et al, 1987) and in T47D human mammary tumor cells (Lamp et al, 1981). There is a markedly enhanced biological potency of the fish hormones (salmon and eel calcitonins) and receptor affinity as compared to calcitonins from other species. The tight, almost irreversible binding of salmon calcitonin to its receptor (a Kd-value of 70 pM was estimated on LLC-PK1 cells; Jans et al 1986) leads to a bypass of cyclase down-regulation processes which is similar to that induced by the covalently binding vasopressin analogue, activation persisting up to 12 h. This is in contrast to human calcitonin, the response to which are rapidly down-regulated in similar fashion to vasopressin (Jans and Hemmings unpublished).

CONCLUSIONS

The molecualar basis of the apparent persistent activation of adenylate cyclase by the activated vasopressin analogue would appear to be the formation of a covalent hormone receptor complex. The covalent linkage of apa-LVP to the V2-receptor through photoactivation prevents dissociation of ligand and receptor either by normal receptor affinity transition induced by receptor phosphorylation or by the low lysosomal pH-value acting on the internalized complex. In this irreversible complex the analogue is presumably in a permanently active conformation.

Concomitant with this bypass of down-regulation processes operating on the V2 receptor is an apparent continuous stimulating signal to the adenylate cyclase, wherby termination of adenylate cyclase activation fails to take place through the normal cellular down-regulation processes. It is possible that the covalent linkage of apa-LVP to the V2 receptor locks the α-subunit of Gs and the catalytic moiety of the adenylate cyclase into a permanently activated form which is then not functional as a target for the down regulatory processes operating at the level of the G-proteins or adenylate cyclase.

PERSPECTIVES

The cytotoxic effect of prolonged stimulation of cAMP production in LLC-PK1 cells induced by the photoactivated vasopressin analogue has been used to select mutants in hormone responsiveness. By this approach we obtained one class of mutants in which all in vivo cAMP mediated responses were reduced (Luzius et al, 1989). Even under conditions of long term stimulation of cAMP production (eg. treatment with the photoactivated vasopressin analogue) in vivo down regulation of the cellular response occurs more quickly or more efficiently in the mutant. The mutant might contain a mutation affecting a key regulation step of cyclase down-regulation. Work is currently under progress to define the exact nature of this mutation. This should lead to a better understanding of the regulatory processes operating on cyclase subsequent to agonist stimulation, which appear to be the processes that are bypassed under conditions of long term stimulation of cyclase exerted by photoactivated vasopressin analogues or salmon calcitonin.

REFERENCES

Benovic, J.L., Bouvier, M., Caron, M.G. and Lefkowitz, R.J. (1988): Regulation of adenylyl cyclase-coupled β-adrenergic receptors: Ann. Rev. Cell. Biol. 4: 405-428.

Dayer, J.M., Vassalli, J.D., Bobbit, J.L., Hull, R.N., Reich, E. and Krane, S.M. (1981): Calcitonin stimulates plasminogen activator in porcine renal tubular cells: LLC-PK1. J. Cell. Biol. 91: 195-200

Eggena, P., Fahrenholz, F. and Schwartz, I.L. (1983): Irreversible stimulation of hydroosmotic response in toad bladder by photoaffinity labelling with Phe2, Phe(p-N3)3 vasopressin. Endocrinology 113: 1413-1421.

Eggena, P., Fahrenholz, F. and Schwartz, I.L. (1984): Covalent linkage of Phe2, Phe(p-N3)3 AVP to vasopressin recpetors in toad bladder during photolysis. Am. J. Physiol. 246: C486-C493.

Elalouf, J-M., Sari, D.C., Roinel, N. and Rouffignac, C. (1988): Desensitization of rat renal thick ascending limb cells to vasopressin. Proc. Natl. Acad. Sci. USA 85: 2407-2411.

Fahrenholz, F. and Crause, C. (1984): 1,6-α-Aminosuberic acid, 3-(p-Azidophenyl-alanine), 8-Arginine vasopressin as a photoaffinity label for renal vasopressin receptors an evaluation. Biochem. Biophys. Res. Commun. 122: 974-982.

Fahrenholz, F., Boer, R., Crause, P. and Tóth, M. (1985): Photoaffinity labelling
   of the renal V2 vasopressin receptor -Identification and enrichment of a
   vasopressin-binding-subunit. Eur. J. Biochem. 152: 589-595.
Fahrenholz, F., Eggena, P., Gazis, D., Tóth, M.V. and Schwartz, I.L. (1986):
   Photoreactive neurohypophyseal hormone analogues: Effects on transport
   processes in mammalian and amphibian epithelia. Endocrinology 118: 1026-1031.
Hemmings, B.A. (1986): cAMP mediated proteolysis of the catalytic subunit of
   cAMP-dependent protein kinase. FEBS LETT. 196: 126-130.
Hull, R.N., Cherry, W.R. and Weaver, G.W. (1976): The origin and characteristics
   of a pig kidney cell strain. In vitro 12: 670-677.
Jans, D.A., Resink, T.J., Wilson, E.R., Reich, E. and Hemmings, B.A. (1986):
   Isolation of a mutant LLC-PK1 cell line defective in hormonal responsiveness: a
   pleiotropic tesion in receptor function. Eur. J. Biochem. 160: 407-412.
Jans, D.A., Gajdas, E.L., Dierks-Ventling C., Hemmings, B.A. and Fahrenholz, F.
   (1987): Long term stimulation of cAMP production in LLC-PK1 pig kidney
   epithelial cells by salmon calcitonin or a photoactivatable analogue of
   vasopressin. Biochim. Biophys. Acta: 930: 392-400.
Kirk, K.L. (1988): Binding and internalization of a fluorescent vasopressin
   analogue by collecting duct cells. Am. J. Physiol.: 255: C622-C632.
Lamp, S.J., Findlay, D.M., Moseley, J.M. and Martin, T.J. (1981) Calcitonin
   induction of a persistent activated state of adenylate cyclase in human breast
   cancer cells (T47D) J. Biol. Chem. 256: 12269-12274.
Lester, B.R., Sheppard, J.R., Burman, M., Somkuti, S.B. and Stassen, F.L. (1985):
   Desensitization of LLC-PK1 cells by vasopressin results in receptor
   down-regulation. Mol. and Cellul. Endocrinology 40: 193-204.
Luzius, H., Jans, D.A. and Fahrenholz, F. (1989) Use of photoactivatable analogue
   of vasopressin to select mutants of the LLC-PK1 porcine kidney cell line
   affected in cAMP-mediated hormonal response. (manuscript in preparation).
Nagamine, Y., Sudol, M. and Reich, E. (1983): Hormonal regulation of plasminogen
   activator mRNA production in porcine kidney cells. Cell 32: 1181-1190.
Rajerison, R., Marchetti, J., Roy, C., Bockaert, J. and Jard, S. (1974): The
   vasopressin-sensitive adenylate cyclase of the rat kidney. J. Biol. Chem. 249,
   6390-6400.
Roy, C., Hall, D., Karish, M. and Ausiello, D.A. (1981): Relationship of
   (8-lysine)vasopressin receptor transition to receptor functional properties
   in a pig kidney cell line (LLC-PK1). J. Biol. Chem. 256: 3423-3427.
Schwartz, J.P. and Passoneau, J.V. (1974): Cyclic-AMP mediated induction of the
   cyclic AMP phosphodiesterase of C-6 glioma cells. Proc. Natl. Acad. Sci. USA
   71: 3844-3848.

Hormones and Cell Regulation. N° 14, Eds J. Nunez, J.E. Dumont. Colloque INSERM/J. Libbey Eurotext Ltd. © 1989. Vol. 198, pp. 27-32

AMPA-sensitive excitatory amino acid receptors in the chick brain

Jeremy M. Henley and Eric A. Barnard

Molecular Neurobiology Unit, Medical Research Council Centre, Hills Road, Cambridge CB2 2QH, England

Excitatory amino acid (EAA) receptors are an abundant neurotransmitter receptor type in the vertebrate central nervous system and are thought to be crucial for many basic functions of the brain. In addition, 'excitotoxic' EAA receptor activation has been implicated in a number of clinically important neuronal disease states including Alzheimer's disease, Huntington's disease and epilepsy (for review see Brehm et al., 1988; Choi, 1988). Since the initial discovery that L-glutamate and L-aspartate depolarise neurones in the mammalian CNS (Curtis et al., 1959; 1960), three main categories of EAA receptor have been established by both electrophysiological and ligand binding studies: the NMDA type, the quisqualate type and the kainate type (Watkins and Evans, 1981; Foster and Fagg, 1984). It is becoming increasingly clear, however, that a heterogeneity of receptor subclasses may exist within each main category. The best documented example of this heterogeneity is the two subclasses of quisqualate receptor, one of which is a second messenger-coupled receptor which stimulates increases in intracellular Ca^{2+} by G protein activation of inositol 1,4,5-triphosphate production (Sladeczek et al., 1985; Nicoletti et al., 1986; Recasens et al., 1987). The other quisqualate receptor subclass is an ionophore-linked receptor, discussed below.

The NMDA receptor is the most extensively studied ionophore-coupled EAA receptor-subtype. Electrophysiological studies have shown that this receptor is associated with an ion channel of large conductance (~50 pS) which is permeable to both Na^+ and Ca^{2+}. The channel is blocked in a voltage-sensitive manner by Mg^{2+}, shows slow desensitisation kinetics, and channel activiation requires the presence of . glycine (for reviews see Mayer and Westbrook, 1987; Krnjevic, 1989). Kainate and quisqualate receptors possess quite different electrophysiological characteristics. These receptor-coupled channels are permeable to Na^+ but not Ca^{2+}, and have main conductance states of <20 pS. The quisqualate receptor, studied using the selective ligand α-amino-3-hydroxy-5-methylisoxazolepropionate (AMPA), shows rapid desensitisation kinetics. The kainate receptor, however, does not desensitise (Mayer and Vyklicky, 1989) and neither of these non-NMDA receptor channels are modulated by Mg^{2+} (Asher and Nowak, 1988). In contrast, comparatively little is known about the biochemistry or molecular structure of these receptors. Recently, however, we have solubilised the binding sites for [^{3}H]kainate and [^{3}H]AMPA with their binding activities intact and with the retention of their pharmacological characteristics.

AMPA is a heterocyclic analogue of L-glutamate related to ibotenic acid which was first synthesised by Krogsgaard-Larsen and coworkers (1980). It is a potent excitant of the cat spinal neurones where the evoked responses are similar to those seen with quisqualate and are not blocked by NMDA receptor antagonists (Krogsgaard-Larsen et al., 1980). Initial [^{3}H]AMPA binding studies were performed on rat cortical membranes (Honore et al., 1982) but a greater density of high affinity [^{3}H]AMPA binding sites has subsequently been found in neuronal membranes from several species of lower vertebrates including goldfish brain (Henley and Oswald, 1988b) and chick brain (Henley and Barnard, 1989b).

In rat brain membranes, [^{3}H]AMPA binding is markedly enhanced in the presence of the chaotrope thiocyanate and Honore and Nielsen (1985) and Murphy et al. (1987) have demonstrated that SCN^- alters the affinity of [^{3}H]AMPA binding without increasing the number of sites (B_{max}). Similarly, in one-day-old chick brain membranes, approximately threefold more [^{3}H]AMPA binding sites are detected in the presence than in the absence of SCN^-.

Chick brain is a good system in which to study EAA receptors for several reasons: the binding sites for each of the EAA receptor subtypes are especially abundant in one-day-old chick brain (Henley and Barnard, 1989b); *Xenopus* oocytes, when injected with mRNA from one-day-old chick brain express more quisqualate and kainate binding sites than oocytes injected with mRNA from any mammalian species (Smart et al., 1986); evidence for a role of EAA receptors in the process of imprinting in the chick, a well defined and quantifiable model for learning and memory in higher vertebrates, has been reported (McCabe and Horn, 1988).

In the presence of 0.1 M KSCN, [^{3}H]AMPA binding to extensively-washed, freeze-thawed membranes from one-day-old chick brain is saturable, with K_D and B_{max} values of 55 nM and 2.6 pmol/mg protein (Henley and Barnard, 1989b). Linear Scatchard plots and Hill coefficients close to unity suggest that [^{3}H]AMPA binds to a single class of sites. The [^{3}H]AMPA binding sites have been solubilised from one-day-old chick brain with their binding activity intact (Henley and Barnard, 1989b) with 1% *N*-octyl-β-D-glucopyranoside (OGP) in the presence of 0.1M KSCN. In the detergent extract, [^{3}H]AMPA bound with a K_D of 69 nM and there was an apparent increase in B_{max} (4.6 pmol/mg protein) compared to the number of sites present in membrane fragments. These results

28

suggest that solubilisation with OGP exposes a pool of 'cryptic' sites which are inaccessible in the membrane fragment preparations.

The association kinetics of [³H]AMPA to OGP solubilised sites are best fitted by a single exponential, but the dissociation kinetics are biphasic with rate constants of 0.117 min⁻¹ and 0.015 min⁻¹. These data suggest the existence of two populations of binding sites, a predominant population (~85%) with a K_D value of 81 nM and a comparatively small population (~15% with a K_D of 2 nM) of higher affinity sites which was not detected by equilibrium binding experiments. The rank order of potency for ligands at displacing [³H]AMPA binding from both membrane-bound and solubilised sites is quisqualate = AMPA > 6-cyano-2,3-dihydroxy-7-nitro-qunioxaline (CNQX) > L-glutamate.

One major aim of our studies is to isolate and purify to homogeneity the AMPA-sensitive quisqualate receptor from one-day-old chick brain; a variety of purification stratergies have been attempted thus far. The solubilised [³H]AMPA binding sites do not elute from an ion-exchange column at a specific NaCl concentration and on sucrose density centrifugation they sediment near to the 60% sucrose cushion at the bottom of the gradient. Inclusion of 1M NaCl in the sucrose density gradients, however, results in a well-defined peak of [³H]AMPA binding activity with a sedimentation coefficient of 9.2S. These results suggest that the binding sites aggregate in solution, but in high-salt gradients, where aggregation is hindered, the sedimentation coefficient is similar to those seen for other putative neuronal EAA receptors including the kainate binding site from·Xenopus (8.6S) (Henley and Barnard, 1989a) and goldfish (8.3S) (Henley and Oswald, 1988a). Significant enrichment of [³H]AMPA binding sites is achieved by wheat germ lectin chromatography, where the specific activity of binding sites is enriched 10-20-fold on elution from the column with 0.3M N-actyl-D-glucosamine (Henley and Barnard, 1989b). We are also investigating affinity-column purification techniques using modified ligands, specific for the AMPA-sensitive quisqualate receptor, which can be immobilised on to a Sepharose support (in collaboration with P. Krogsgaard-Larsen, Copenhagen).

In parallel with these purification attempts, we are further characterising the properties of the membrane-bound and solubilised binding sites. One technique we have utilised is target size analysis. This method allows the molecular weight of proteins to be estimated from the dose of ionising radiation needed to inactivate them (Kepner and Macey, 1968; Neilsen and Braestrup, 1988). Radiation inactivation of the [³H]AMPA binding to chick telencephalon (Henley, Neilsen and Barnard, unpublished) yield qualitatively similar results to those reported for rat cortex (Honore and Nielsen, 1985). In both rat and chick brain tissues, a complex curvilinear inactivation plot is generated when the natural log of the residual binding activity is plotted against the radiation dose. These data suggest the existence of a large molecular weight modulatory component associated with the binding subunit. This modulatory component down-regulates the affinity of the binding subunit for [³H]AMPA. As the modulatory component is inactivated by high energy radiation, the affinity of [3H]AMPA binding is increased thus causing an apparent increase in binding sites determined with a single [3H]AMPA concentration. The estimated molecular weights are approximately 62,000 for the binding subunit and 134,000 for the modulatory component in chick brain.

We have also investigated the anatomical distribution of [3H]AMPA and other glutamatergic ligand binding sites in the one-day-old chick brain by quantitative autoradiography (Henley et al., 1989). As seen in the rat (Monaghan et al., 1984; Rainbow et al., 1984), the chick hippocampal areas possess the highest density of [3H]AMPA binding. Elsewhere in the chick telencephalon the distribution of [3H]AMPA binding sites is relatively uniform, although the neostriatum has a marginally higher density of sites than other striatal areas. The density of [3H]AMPA binding sites in the diencephalon is comparatively low, with the highest concentration of sites occurring in the thalamus. In the optic lobes the striatum griseum et fibrosum superficiale is well defined by [3H]AMPA and in the cerebellum [3H]AMPA binding is more dense in the molecular layer than in the granule cell layer.

Although the identity of the endogenous ligand(s) for quisqualate receptors, and the precise neurophysiological functions mediated by these proteins, remain unclear, the elucidation of the role of quisqualate and other EAA receptors in neuronal function and in the aetiology of neurodegenerative diseases is seen as a goal of major importance.

This work was supported by the Medical Research Council.

References.

Ascher, P. and Nowak, L. (1988) Quisqualate- and kainate-activated channels in mouse central neurones in culture. J. Physiol. 399, 227-245.
Brehm, I, L., Jorgensen, F.S., Hansen, J.J. and Krogsgaard-Larsen, P. (1988) Agonists and antagonists for central glutamic acid receptors. Drug News Perpectives. 1, 138-144.
Choi, D.W. (1988) Glutamate neurotoxicity and diseases of the nervous system. Neuron. 1, 623-634.
Curtis, D.R., Phillis, J.W. and Watkins, J.C. (1959) Chemical excitation of spinal neurones. Nature. 183, 611.
Curtis, D.R., Phillis, J.W. and Watkins, J.C. (1960) The excitation of spinal neurones by certain acidic amino acids. J. Physiol. Lond. 150, 656-682.
Foster, A.C. and Fagg, G.E. (1984) Acidic amino acid binding sites in mammalian neuronal membranes: their characteristics and relationship to synaptic receptors. Brain Res. Rev. 7, 103-164.
Henley, J.M. and Oswald, R.E. (1988a) Solubilisation and characterisation of kainate binding sites from goldfish brain. Biochem. Biophys. Acta. 937, 102-111.

Henley, J.M. and Oswald, R.E. (1988b) Characterisation and regional distribution of glutamatergic and cholinergic ligand binding sites in goldfish brain. J. Neurosci. 8, 2101-2107.

Henley, J.M. and Barnard, E.A. (1989a) Kainate receptors in *Xenopus* central nervous system: solubilisation with n-octyl-β-D-glucopyranoside. J. Neurochem. 52, 31-37.

Henley, J.M. and Barnard, E.A. (1989b) Solubilisation and characterisation of a putative quisqualate-type glutamate receptor from chick brain. J. Neurochem. in press.

Henley, J.M., Moratalla, R., Hunt, S.P. and Barnard, E.A. (1989) Localisation and quantitative autoradiography of glutamatergic ligand binding sites in chick brain. Eur. J. Neurosci. in press.

Honore, T. (1989) Excitatory amino acid receptor subtypes and specific antagonists. Med. Res. Rev. 9, 1-23.

Honore, T., Lauridsen, J. and Krogsgaard-Larsen, P. (1982) The binding of [3H]AMPA, a structural analogue of glutamic acid, to rat brain membranes. J. Neurochem. 38, 173-178.

Honore, T. and Nielsen, M. (1985) Complex structure of quisqualate-sensitive glutamate receptors in rat cortex. Neurosci. Lett. 54, 27-32.

Kepner, G.R. and Macey, R.I. (1968) Membrane enzyme systems: Molecular size determination by radiation inactivation. Biochem. Biophys. Acta. 163, 188-203.

Krnjevic, K. (1988) Electrophysiology of excitatory amino acids. in Allosteric modulation of amino acid receptors: Therapeutic implications. Vol. 1 pp. 209-224. Eds. E.A. Barnard and E. Costa.

Krogsgaard-Larsen, P., Honore, T., Hansen, J.J., Curtis, D.R. and Lodge, D. (1980) A new class of glutamate agonist structurally related to ibotenic acid. Nature (London) 284, 64-66.

Mayer, M.L. and Westbrook, G.L. (1987) The physiology of excitatory amino acids in the vertebrate central nervous system. Prog. Neurobiol. 28, 197-276.

Mayer, M.L. and Vyklicky, L. (1989) Concanavalin A selectively reduces desensitistaion of mammalian neuronal quisqualate receptors. Proc. Natl. Acad. Sci. USA. 86, 1411-1415.

McCabe, B. and Horn, G. (1988) Learning and memory: Regional changes in NMDA receptors in the chick brain after imprinting Proc. Natl. Acad. Sci. USA. 85, 2849-2853.

Monaghan, D.T., Yao, D. and Cotman, C.W. (1984) Distribution of [3H]AMPA binding sites in rat brain as determined by quantitative autoradiography. Brain Res. 324, 160-164.

Murphy, D.E., Snowhill, E.W. and Williams, M. (1987) Characterisation of quisqualate recognition sites in rat brain tissue using [3H]AMPA and a filtration binding assay. Neurochem. Res. 187, 113-127.

Nicoletti, F., Meek, J.L., Iadarola, M., Chuang, D.M., Roth, B.L. and Costa, E. (1986) Coupling of inositol phospholipid metabolism with excitatory amino acid recognition sites in rat hippocampus. J. Neurochem. 46, 40-46.

Nielsen, M. and Braestrup, C. (1988) The apparent target size of rat brain benzodiazepine receptor, acetylcholinesterase and pyruvate kinase is highly influenced by experimental conditions. J. Biol. Chem. 24, 11900-11906.

Olsen, R.W., Szamraj, O. and Houser, C.R. (1987) [3H]AMPA binding to glutamate receptor subpopulations in rat brain. Brain Res. 402, 243-254.

Recasens, M., Sassetti, I., Nourigat, A., Sladeczek, F. and Bockaert, J. (1987) Characterisation of subtypes of excitatory amino acid receptors involved in the stimulation of inositol phosphate synthesis in rat brain synaptoneurosomes. Eor. J. Pharmacol. 414, 87-93.

Rainbow, T.C., Wieczorek, C.M. and Halpain, S. (1984) Quantitative autoradiography of binding sites for [3H]AMPA a structural analogue of glutamic acid. Brain Res. 309, 173-177.

Sladeczek, F., Pin, J.P., Recasens, M., Bockaert, J. and Weiss, S. (1985) Glutamate stimulates inositol phosphate formation in striatal neurones. Nature. 317, 717-719.

Smart, T.G., Constanti, G., Bilbe, D.A., Brown, D.A., Barnard, E.A. and Van Renterghem, C. (1986) Expression of vertebrate amino acid receptors in *Xenopus* oocytes. Adv. Expl. Med. Biol. 203, 525-537.

Watkins, J.C. and Evans, R.H. (1981) Excitatory amino acid transmitters. Annu. Rev. Pharmacol. Toxicol. 21, 165-204.

Hormones and Cell Regulation. N° 14, Eds J. Nunez, J.E. Dumont. Colloque INSERM/J. Libbey Eurotext Ltd. © 1989. Vol. 198, pp. 33-36

Homology cloning of cDNAs amplified by the polymerase chain reaction. Identification of four new members of the G-protein coupled receptor family

Frédérick Libert, Marc Parmentier, Anne Lefort, Christiane Dinsart, Jacqueline Van Sande, Carine Maenhaut, Marie-Jeanne Simons, Jacques E. Dumont and Gilbert Vassart*

*Institut de Recherche Interdisciplinaire, Faculté de Médecine, Université Libre de Bruxelles, Campus Erasme, 808 route de Lennik, 1070 Bruxelles, and *Service de Génétique Médicale, Secteur de génétique moléculaire, Université Libre de Bruxelles, Hôpital Erasme, 808 route de Lennik, 1070 Bruxelles, Belgique*

SUMMARY

A strategy for homology cloning exploiting the polymerase chain reaction has been devised to clone new members of the family of genes encoding G protein-coupled receptors. It involves the use of "degenerated" primers corresponding to sequences of the third and sixth transmembrane segments of known receptors belonging to this gene family. Clones encoding three known receptors and four new putative receptors were thus obtained from thyroid cDNA. Sequence similarity between one of the putative receptors and the 5HT1a receptor was observed, suggesting that it could be a member of the large serotonergic receptors. Expression of the receptor cDNAs in microinjected, or transfected cells, should allow identification of the corresponding ligands.

Cloning and sequencing of the β_2 adrenergic receptor has demonstrated that it is evolutionary related to the visual pigment opsin (Dixon et al., 1986). This led to the identification of a number of receptors constituting a new gene family which have in common the presence of seven transmembrane segments and the ability to interact with G proteins. With the aim to clone the thyrotropin receptor, we have devised a strategy based on the polymerase chain reaction (PCR) (Saiki et al., 1988) to amplify and clone cDNAs belonging to this gene family. Using primers corresponding to consensus sequences of the third and sixth transmembrane segments of available receptors, we have cloned three known and four new members of this gene family that are expressed in thyroid tissue (Libert et al., 1989).

Poly(A)-rich RNA prepared from human thyroid tissue was reverse transcribed and the resulting cDNAs were subjected to amplification by PCR using a set of highly "degenerated" primers. These were devised from the analysis of sequences corresponding to the third and sixth

transmembrane segments of the following receptors: beta 1,
beta 2 and alpha 2 adrenergic receptors (Frielle et al.,
1987; Kobilka et al., 1987; Kobilka et al., 1987); M1
muscarinic receptor (Kubo et al., 1986); substance K
receptor (Masu et al., 1987) and 5HT1a (Kobilka et al.,
1987; Fargin et al., 1988). The sequence similarity
between the different receptors in these segments was
around 65%. Each primer consisted of a mixture of
oligonucleotides with a number of degeneracies allowing a
78% match, or better, with any receptors in the list. The
primer composition was oriented arbitrarily towards 1-,
2-adrenergic and the 5HT1a receptors in order to avoid
excessive degeneracy.

After 55 PCR cycles, a pattern of discrete cDNA species was
observed by agarose gel electrophoresis. Individual cDNAs
were cloned in M13 bacteriophage derivatives and
sequenced. Out of 80 clones analysed, 40 contained
sequences with a strong similarity with receptors coupled
to G proteins. These were classified into seven
categories: five corresponded to sequences encoding unknown
receptors and two contained the sequences of the β_2
adrenergic and the 5HT1a receptors. Considering the
expected scarcity of the corresponding mRNAs in the thyroid
tissue, the proportion of clones with the characteristics
of receptors gives a measure of the extraordinary
enrichment achieved by the procedure.

The complete primary structure of the putative receptors
was determined from full-length clones isolated from a
lambda gt11 cDNA library of dog thyroid. They were termed
RDC1, RDC4, RDC5, RDC7 and RDC8, respectively. The dog and
human sequences were more than 90% similar in the region
between transmembrane segments III and VI for which comparison was available. From the alignment of the candidate
receptors with the sequence of the β_2 receptor, taken as
the archetype, overwhelming evidence was obtained that they
all belong to the same multi-gene superfamily. This conclusion is supported by the fact that the hamster $\alpha 1$ adrenergic sequence, which became available while sequencing of
our clones was in progress (Cotecchia et al., 1988), is 91%
identical to that of clone RDC5. We therefore consider
RDC5 to represent the dog α_1 receptor.

The similarities between the known and newly isolated
potential receptors were computed. RDC4 appears related to
the 5HT1a receptor while RDC7 is closer to RDC8 than to any
of the others. Besides their high homology, RDC7 and RDC8
both display a very short N-terminal extracellular domain
which is devoid of potential N-glycosylation sites. This
makes them members of a new subfamily in the G protein
coupled receptors. The last potential receptor, RDC1, is
clearly different from all other receptors. If anything,
it resembles somewhat substance K receptor. The nature of
the ligands of these new candidate receptors remains an
open question. The similarity of RDC4 with 5HT1a suggests
that it could be a member of the large family of serotonin
receptors (Peroutka, 1988). However, only functional and/

or binding assays will allow to identify them correctly. Tissue distribution of the candidate receptors was investigated by Northern blotting. Poly(A) RNA from nine dog tissues were investigated. None of the transcripts displayed the thyroid specificity expected for the TSH receptor; each probe hybridized to RNA from a different selection of tissues. RDC7 and RDC8 were both expressed in the brain, with RDC7 transcripts being also present in the thyroid. RDC1 transcripts were clearly found in the heart, kidney and thyroid. RDC5 (the dog α_1-adrenergic receptor) was present in most tissues tested, except the thyroid. RDC4 gave virtually no signal on the blot with RNA from any tissue. The observation that transcripts of RDC4, RDC5 and RDC8 could barely be detected in the thyroid, suggests that the amplification and selectivity of the procedure lead to the cloning of receptors belonging to minor cell populations present in the thyroid gland.

The use of the PCR method with a set of degenerated primers is clearly superior to homology cloning methods based on the screening of libraries with cross-hybridizing probes. The amplification and selectivity achieved yield a low cloning background compatible with the direct identification of clones by DNA sequencing. Selection of the primer sequences and degeneracies should allow to target amplification towards subfamilies of genes. The method should be generally applicable to the study of multigene families as well as to the cloning of homologous genes in different species.

ACKNOWLEDGMENTS

We are thankful to P. Cochaux, C. Christophe and S. Swillens for help with PCR, oligonucleotide synthesis and the handling of data banks, respectively. Supported by grants from Ministère de la Politique Scientifique, FRSM, NIH, Solvay SA and Association Recherche Biomédicale et Diagnostic asbl. F.L., C.M. are fellows from IRSIA; M.P. was chargé de Recherche at the FNRS.

REFERENCES

Cotecchia, S. et al., (1988) Proc. Natl. Acad. Sci. USA 85, 7159-7163.
Dixon, R.A.F. et al., (1986) Nature 321, 75-79.
Fargin, A. et al., (1988) Nature 335, 358-360.
Frielle, T. et al., (1987) Proc. Natl. Acad. Sci. USA 84, 7920-7924.
Kobilka, B.K. et al., (1987) Science 238, 650-656.
Kobilka, B.K. et al., (1987) Nature 329, 75-79.
Kobilka, B.K. et al., (1987) Proc. Natl. Acad. Sci. USA 84, 46-50.
Kubo, T. et al., (1986) Nature 323, 411-416.
Libert, F. et al., (1989) Science 22, 569-572.
Masu, Y. et al., (1987) Nature 329, 836-838.
Peroutka, S.J. (1988) TINS 11, 496-500.
Saiki, R.K. et al., (1988) Science 239, 487-491.

Résumé

Une stratégie basée sur la réaction en chaîne de la polymérase (PCR) a été mise au point pour cloner de nouveaux membres de la famille des récepteurs couplés à des protéines G. La méthode utilise un couple d'amorces "dégénérées" correspondant aux séquences des zones transmembranaires n° 3 et n° 6 d'une série de récepteurs dont la séquence est connue. Appliquée au tissu thyroïdien, cette approche a permis le clonage de trois récepteurs déjà connus et de quatre nouveaux candidats récepteurs dont l'un présente une similitude de séquence avec le récepteur sérotonergique 5HT1a. L'expression des cDNAs de ces nouveaux récepteurs dans des systèmes d'expression devrait permettre l'identification des ligands correspondants.

Regulation of gene expression

Régulation de l'expression génique

Hormones and Cell Regulation. N° 14, Eds J. Nunez, J.E. Dumont. Colloque INSERM/J. Libbey Eurotext Ltd. © 1989. Vol. 198, pp. 39-44

Promoter and enhancer activation properties of the glucocorticoid receptor

Michael Schatt, Stefan Wieland and Sandro Rusconi

Institut für Molekularbiologie II der Universität Zürich, Hönggerberg ETH-HPM, CH-8093 Zürich, Switzerland.

Steroid hormone receptors are modular regulatory proteins which exert their genomic effects by binding to specific target sites on the DNA (for a review, see **Beato, 1989**). The target sites are found at variable distance from the transcription initiation region and are named after the corresponding regulator (i. e the acronym GRE denotes a Glucocorticoid Response Element.). Several lines of evidence have suggested that the binding of the DNA target sites occurs only after activation of the receptor by the specific ligand. The process of activation is yet poorly understood and it might involve the direct interaction of the hormone binding domain with other proteins such as the heat shock protein 90 (**Pratt et al., 1988**). In the case of the Glucocorticoid Receptor (GR), the deletion of the hormone binding domain (rat GR residues ~ 550-795 , (**Godowski et al., 1987**)) leads to a truncated receptor fragment which exhibits all the properties of a strong, still GRE-specific and constitutive (= hormone-independent) transcription factor (**Godowski et al., 1987; Rusconi & Yamamoto, 1987**) (see also below). Recent reports have also suggested that the GR can cooperate with a whole array of ubiquitous transcription factors to activate promoters in an apparent synergistic manner (**Schüle et al., 1988**). In these experiments the distance between the GRE and the target site for the cooperating factor was relatively small and the combined sites were placed in proximity of the transcription start. In this situation it is very difficult to distinguish between direct and indirect modes of cooperation. In particular, one could speculate that the observed synergism is due to mutual help in displacing an inhibitory competitor such as a nucleosome (**Beato, 1989**). This rather indirect type of cooperation might be invoked to explain a number of apparent synergisms occurring within a promoter, but would certainly be insufficient to explain the cooperation between an enhancer and a promoter.

RESULTS AND DISCUSSION

With these questions in mind, we have constructed a series of rabbit β–globin reporter genes (see **Fig. 1**) in which an increasing number of palindromic GREs (symbolized by the letter "P") is placed either in proximity of the TATA-box (= promoter position, see P1-β, P2-β and P4-β) or at 2 kb distance (downstream = enhancer position, see β–P4 in **Fig. 1**). We also generated reporter genes in which the P4 at enhancer position is combined with either one palindromic GRE at promoter position (see P1-β-P4) or with other ubiquitous factor binding sites close to the TATA-box (see the general scheme of XY-β-P4). The aim of this last series was to assess, whether the GRE-based enhancer (called P4) would manifest any preference for a particular promoter configuration. Each reporter gene was transiently expressed in HeLa cells, either alone or in the presence of a co-transfected effector plasmid encoding a specific GR fragment. The comparison of the globin RNA levels obtained in presence of the activator with the signal obtained in its absence gave the specific stimulation of each reporter gene as shown in **Table 1**. The major conclusions which could be drawn from these co-transfection assays are listed below.

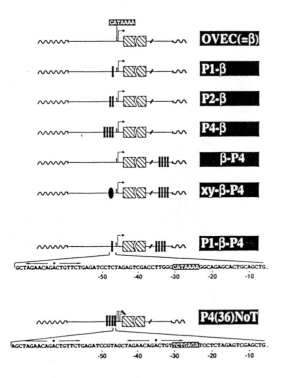

FIGURE 1. GR regulated reporter genes.

The reporter genes are based on the OVEC rabbit β–globin vector described by Westin et al. (1987). Hyphenated Palindromic GREs (Severne et al., 1988) were placed at the indicated position (black rectangles) with respect to the transcription initiation site (flag with arrow). In the multimeric clusters the distance between palindrome centres is 28 bp. The clusters at enhancer position were placed 1.8 kb downstream (Xba site, Westin et al., 1987). Sequence details at bottom show a TATA-box containing promoter (in the case of P1-β-P4) and one example of a TATA-depleted promoter in which the most proximal palindromic GRE is placed 36 bp upstream of initiation (construct P4-(36)NoT).In other TATA-less constructions the centre of the most proximal GRE was at different positions (see results in FIG. 2). Other symbols: wavy line, plasmid sequences; thin line, flanking beta globin genomic sequences; Hatched box, globin gene coding region, Arrows above sequence, palindromic GREs; numbers below sequence, position relative to natural initiation site; XY and filled oval denote anyone of the binding sites for the ubiquitous transcription factors listed in Table 1.

Synergism at the promoter position.

There is a non-linear relationship between the number of GRE targets at the promoter and the level of stimulation by the constitutive GR fragment GR3-556 (see samples 1 to 4 in **Table 1**). In fact, the increase from 0, to 1, to 2 and to 4 GREs results in a 0, <10, >50 and >1000 fold stimulation, respectively. This indicates that even "strong" GREs can exhibit a marked tendency to work synergistically when placed at the appropriate distance to each other. This cooperative behaviour had been suggested previously to be a prerogative of "weak" (= imperfect) GREs (**Beato, 1989** and references therein). We suggest that this synergistic behaviour might derive from the combination of both, the mutual facilitation of binding by i.e. displacing a competing nucleosome, together with a stabilization of otherwise weak protein-protein interactions which could occur between the bound GR and the transcriptional machinery. In the course of these experiments, we noticed that the wild type GR does not show a similar synergistic behaviour with the increasing number of tightly spaced palindromic

GREs (**Wieland et al., 1988**). Recent experiments (data not shown) seem to suggest that this is simply due to the large size of the intact receptor which probably cannot fully occupy the P4 cluster.

TABLE 1. Promoter and enhancer stimulation by GR fragments.

NR	REPORTER GENE		TRANSACTIVATOR	STIMULATION
	promoter	enhancer	GR fragment	stim. / unstim.
1	NONE	NONE	GR 3-556	1
2	P1	NONE	GR 3-556	10X
3	P2	NONE	GR 3-556	>50X
4	P4	NONE	GR 3-556	>1000X
5	NONE	P4	GR 3-556	>30X
6	P1	P4	GR 3-556	>300X
7	XY	NONE	GR 3-556	1
8	SP1	P4	GR 3-556	>20X
9	OCT.U	P4	GR 3-556	>15X
10	OCT.B	P4	GR 3-556	>15X
11	MRE	P4	GR 3-556	>30X
12	P1	NONE	GR-407-556	<2X
13	P2	NONE	GR-407-556	>20X
14	P4	NONE	GR-407-556	>50X
15	P1	P4	GR-407-556	>40X
16	P1	NONE	GAL-407-556-GC	<5X
17	P2	NONE	GAL-407-556-GC	>30X
18	P4	NONE	GAL-407-556-GC	>500X
19	P1	P4	GAL-407-556-GC	>150X

The reporter genes (see Fig. 1 for structural details) were co-transfected in HeLa cells along with a reference gene (Westin et al, 1987) and either with or without co-transfected effector plasmid encoding the activator (see the column marked TRANSACTIVATOR). The Globin transcripts were detected by S1-nuclease analysis and the signals were evaluated by scintillation counting of the corresponding bands from dried gels and corrected for fluctuations by comparison to the corresponding reference signal. The stimulation (rightmost column) is defined as: corrected signal obtained in presence of activator divided by the corrected signal obtained in absence of activator. Basal levels were mostly undetectable, so that we could only give minimal/maximal values for some constructs. Basal level of Sp1 site containing promoter was detectable and the stimulation could be calculated more precisely. Other symbols: XY, any one of the ubiquitous factor sites (SP1, OCT.B etc); Oct.U and OCT.B, binding sites responding to ubiquitous, respectively B-cell specific octamer binding factor (Müller et al, 1988); MRE, metal response element (Westin et al 1987). Transfection conditions were as described in Severne et al., 1988.

Testing the GR as a "pure" enhancer activating factor.

By displacing the P4 element 2 kb downstream of the transcription initiation site (see β-P4 and XY-β-P4 of Fig. 1). we can virtually exclude that a stimulatory effect could arise from an indirect cooperation such as a mere nucleosome displacement. In the case of β-P4 or P1-β-P4 the molecular distance between the enhancer and the promoter region is about 700 nm along the DNA fibre and about 100 nm along a chromatin fibre. This distance cannot be easily bridged with a simple protein-protein interaction if the fibre is not bent or looped (looping model), or without significant displacement of interacting trans-elements (scanning or diffusion model). We observed that the GR fragment GR3-556 is able to significantly activate transcription, even when forced to bind at this remote position (see sample 5 in Table 1). No other known upstream elements seem to be necessary for this stimulation (β-P4 has a promoter consisting only of the TATA-box, directly linked to position -400, which contains no known transcription factor binding sites (**Westin et al., 1987**)). Furthermore, the addition of a known binding site such as "SP1" or "Octamer" near to the TATA-box (see samples 7-10 in Table 1) does not prevent the stimulation by GR 3-556 although it may increase the basal level (transcription in absence of GR3-556, see legend to Table 1). In fact, the GR-mediated stimulation of each individual XY-β-P4 construct (XY indicates anyone of the above mentioned sites for ubiquitous transcription factors) is approximately the same as the stimulation brought about by an SV40 enhancer placed at the same +2 kb position (M.S., unpublished results). From this, we conclude that the strong interaction between the GR3-556 and the P4 element generates a very powerful enhancer which can stimulate virtually any type of promoter (i.e. consisting of the most disparate variety of factor binding sites).

Domain deletion analysis does not allow the distinction between promoter and enhancer activating function.

One might have expected that further mutation of the GR could generate some GR fragments which have lost the long range stimulation property (i.e. P1-β-P4, see Table 1), while maintaining the capacity of activating transcription from a promoter position (i.e P4-β, see Table 1). Somewhat to our surprise, we could truncate the GR to its essential DNA binding domain and few surrounding aminoacids (GR407-556, **Miesfeld et al., 1987**) and still observe its capacity of stimulating transcription from an enhancer position. This is illustrated by the samples 12-19 of **Table 1**. By combining the effector plasmids encoding either the GR407-556 fragment (samples 12-15), or a "reinforced" chimaera thereof (GAL-407-556-GC, samples 16-19) with the various reporter plasmids, we could demonstrate that these GR fragments display weaker, but qualitatively identical, stimulatory properties when compared to the strong fragment GR3-556 (see samples 2 to 6). This suggests that the residues 3-405 (which are deleted in the mutant GR407-556) might have only an accessory function (at least under the tested conditions) and that the primary requirements for a minimal enhancer activation property must reside within the boundaries 407 to 556. It remains to be seen, whether further deletion or point mutagenesis might allow the distinction of sub-domains (or even single aminoacids) which are indispensable for long range activation properties, while being dispensable for, i.e. promoter activation properties.

GR transcription stimulation does not require the presence of a TATA-box: direct interaction of bound GR with RNA-polymerase ?

We could show that the GR fragment 3-556 behaves as a general enhancer activating protein, but the question remained: does the GR require the presence of general transcription factors such as the TATA-box binding factor in order to exert its transcription stimulatory activity? A recent report for the yeast activator GCN4 suggested that this protein might directly interact with the RNA polymerase, thereby obviating the requirement of a TATA-box (**Chen and Struhl, 1989**). One must however recognize that in yeast the position of the TATA-box with respect to the initiation site is not as tightly conserved as in higher eucaryotes. We therefore wanted to test, whether the depletion of the TATA-box from the rabbit beta globin gene would still permit the stimulation of transcription from the normal initiation site. We constructed several TATA-less promoters in which the most proximal GRE was placed at various distances from the transcription start (see example for position -36 for the most proximal GRE palindrome centre in Fig. 1). These constructs were tested in HeLa cells in absence /presence of the activator GR3-556 (see **Fig 2**). The S1-analysis showed no detectable signal in absence of the activator (see example in lane 1, **Fig. 2a**) but a variety of discrete RNA products whose 5' seems to map at defined positions between +1 and +20 (see lanes 3,4 and 5 in Fig. 2a). We interpret this finding as a possible evidence for the existence of a dominant "initiation box" in the rabbit beta globin gene. We speculate that in the absence of a "framing" activity (such as the one provided by a TATA-box binding factor) the RNA polymerase will still prefer to start transcription within this region, although in a scattered manner, i. e. by generating several discrete 5' ends. This transcription seems to be directly stimulated by the presence of a strong activator (see above) and the choice of specific positions within the initiation cluster seems to depend from the relative position of the most proximal stimulatory factor. This is best illustrated by the densitometric analysis of the radiograms presented in **Fig 2b**. It is evident, for instance, that the relative frequency by which the appearance of discrete downstream start sites in the region +10 to +20 (areas E and F) <u>decreases</u> when the most proximal GRE is shifted from -32 to -48 (compare densitometric profiles of experiments Nr 3 to Nr 5 in **Fig. 2b**). The opposite effect is noticed in the case of the more "natural" sites in the areas A and B (start sites at position +1 to +3). This indicates that the position and orientation of the bound GR has a direct influence on the choice of initiation sites within a cluster (i. e. a closer bound GR induces more downstream start sites and, vice versa, a more remote GR leads to the preference of more upstream positions). We conclude from this that the GR either directly contacts RNA polymerase, or that this contact is mediated by factors which do not have a cis-requirement (i.e. do not have a specific DNA target). Experiments are in progress to determine, whether these effects can be seen also in vitro and whether further displacements of the GR binding site might lead to a construct which has the same preference for the +1 transcription initiation as in the case of the TATA-box containing reporter gene (see control experiment Nr 2).

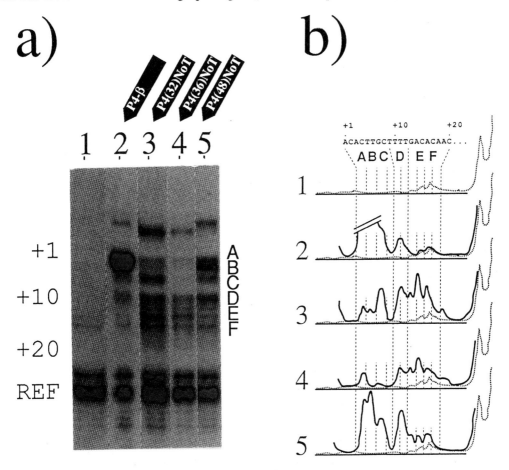

FIGURE 2. GR stimulates Transcription in a TATA-box depleted promoter.

Reporter genes containing a TATA-box (see experiments Nr 1 and 2) or in which the TATA-box had been deleted (experiments Nr1, Nr3, Nr4 and Nr5) were tested in HeLa cells in absence (see experiment Nr1) or in presence of activator (vector producing GR 3-556 added in all other experiments). Specific signals were detected by S1-analysis. **2a**, Panel showing the radiograms. +1, +10, +20 and REF indicate the migration of S1-protected fragments (REF is the position of the mixed-in internal standard (Westin et al., 1987) which yields RNA starting at +29). The lanes: 1, mixed P4-ß and P4(36)NoT in the absence of stimulator; 2, P4-ß in the presence of GR3-556; 3,4 and 5 are the signals obtained from, respectively, P4(32)NoT, P4(36)NoT and P4(48)NoT in presence of stimulator (bracketed numbers indicate the distance between the centre of the most proximal palindromic GRE and the natural transcription site, relevant sequence in the example of P4(36)NoT is given in Fig. 1). **2b** Densitometric evaluation of radiogram presented in 2a. Elerctrophoresis direction is from right to left. Areas A through F correspond to the same regions of the radiogram shown in 2a. Numbers at left indicate the corresponding lane in 2a. On top, the DNA sequence immediately downstream of the initiation site

PERSPECTIVES

The strong activation of the P4-β reporter gene by the GR3-556 fragment let us envisage the possibility of studying the phenomenon in cell-free transcribing extracts. In particular, we are interested in seeing whether the P4 enhancer will also work from a remote position in vitro. To this purpose we are expressing a modified version of the GR 3-556 fragment in bacteria. Preliminary results (U. Döbbeling, unpublished) indicate that this bacterially synthesized GR fragment can specifically bind DNA. The knowledge that the P4 element seems to behave as a general enhancer let us hope that the in vitro study of the GR mediated transcriptional stimulation will provide some useful information for establishing more general models of enhancer function. One striking observation is that the "essential" GR fragment 407-556 is sufficient for activation from a distance, thus implying that the information for enhancer activation must be contained within this relatively short peptide. Other transcription factors, such as the octamer binding factor 2A (**Müller et al., 1988;** W Schaffner, pers. comm.) seem incapable of a similar long range activity even in their intact form. We are trying to verify whether this property can be transferred from the GR to these factors by constructing the appropriate chimaeras. If this is possible, it would mean that the capability of acting from a proximal or a distal location are separable functions which may derive from distinguishable protein:protein contacts. The identification of these specific contacts might give a satisfactory answer to the long standing question regarding the relationships and differences between promoters and enhancers.

LITERATURE CITED

-**Beato M.** (1989). *Cell* **56**, 335-344
-**Chen W. and Struhl K.** (1989). *EMBO J.* **8**, 261-268
-**Godowski P. et al.** (1987). *Nature* **325**, 365-368
-**Miesfeld R. et al.** (1987). *Science* **236**, 423 427
-**Müller M. et al.** (1988). *Nature* **336**, 544-551
-**Pratt W.B. et al.** (1988). *Jour. Biol. Chem.* **263**, 267-273
-**Rusconi S. and Yamamoto K.R.** (1987). *EMBO J.* **6**, 1309-1315
-**Schüle R. et al.** (1988) *Science* **242**, 1418-1420
-**Severne et al.** (1988). *EMBO J.* **7**, 2503-2508
-**Westin G. et al.** (1987). *Nucl. Acids Res.* **15**, 6787-6798
-**Wieland S. et al.** (1988).in: *Molecular Mechanisms and Consequences of activation of Hormone and Growth Factor Receptors.* Ed. CE Sekeris, NATO ASI Series, 1988, in press

Correspondence to be mailed to SR, Institut für Molekularbiologie II, Hönggerberg HPM, CH-8093 Zürich, Switzerland
We would like to thank Professor W. Schaffner for support and "enhancing" discussions, Mrs. Hug for excellent technical assistance; Mr. Ochsenbein for expert contribution in the assembly of figures. This work has been supported by the Kanton Zürich and the Schweizerische Nationalfonds.

Hormones and Cell Regulation. N° 14, Eds J. Nunez, J.E. Dumont. Colloque INSERM/J. Libbey Eurotext Ltd. © 1989. Vol. 198, pp. 45-47

Transcriptional regulation of the tyrosine amino-transferase gene : structure of a regulatory switch

Michael Boshart, Falk Weih, Andrea Schmidt, Doris Nitsch, Francis Stewart and Günther Schütz

Institute of Cell and Tumor Biology, German Cancer Research Center, Im Neuenheimer Feld 280, D-6900 Heidelberg, FRG

INTRODUCTION

To understand the differentiation processes which yield the various cellular phenotypes, it is necessary to elucidate mechanisms by which genes are selectively expressed. Of particular importance for the establishment of a given pattern of gene activity is the interplay between controlling genes and signaling molecules such as hormones. Furthermore, it seems clear that tissue-specific patterns of gene activity depend on both positive and negative regulatory factors. The tyrosine aminotransferase (TAT) gene is an example of a gene whose expression is controlled by positive and negative factors and by hormones. TAT expression is regulated not only by glucocorticoids and by the peptide hormone glucagon acting via the cAMP pathway, but also by two genetically defined, trans-acting loci (Fig. 1).

First, a dominant negative regulator, termed tissue-specific extinguisher (Tse-1), has been defined by intertypic somatic cell hybrids and mapped to a small region of human chromosome 17 (Killary and Fournier, 1984; Lem et al. 1989).

Second, a positive regulator has been postulated to account for the lethal pheno-type of certain albino mice carrying a homozygous deletion around the albino locus on chromosome 7. TAT as well as several other liver-specific enzymes are not expressed in the liver of these newborn albino mice (Gluecksohn-Waelsch, 1979). Since the structural gene for TAT is not deleted, and has been mapped to a chromosome other than 7, it has been suggested that the deletion at the albino locus removes a regulatory locus (Schmid et al., 1985).

Previously, we have shown that glucocorticoid responsiveness of TAT expression is confered by a conditional enhancer 2500 bp upstream of the transcription start site (Jantzen et al., 1987). Here we show that a liver-specific enhancer even further upstream of the TAT promoter, mediates the effect of the dominant negative regulator Tse-1 as well as responsiveness to cAMP. This enhancer has structural and functional characteristics of a signal transducer and we suggest that it works as a regulatory switch which controls the hormone triggered timed onset of expression of the TAT gene in the newborn liver.

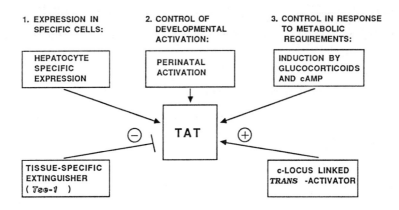

Fig. 1 Control of TAT gene expression

RESULTS AND DISCUSSION

To identify cis-acting sequences mediating the complex transcriptional
regulation of the TAT gene, we fused the TAT promoter including different
portions of its 5'-flanking region to the universal reporter gene chlor-
amphenicol acetyltransferase (CAT) and transiently transfected these constructs
into various cell lines. First, we found that a sequence 3600 bp upstream of the
transcription start site strongly activated CAT expression in well differentiated rat hepatoma cells (FTO2B) but not in rat fibroblasts. A series of
5'- and 3'-deletion mutants defined a sequence of 80 bp absolutely essential for
transcriptional stimulation. This sequence confered hepatoma-specific activation
to the heterologous TK promoter. The same sequence also mediated response to
hormonal signals transduced via the cAMP pathway. We also investigated whether
this sequence was the target for dominant negative regulation by the product of
the tissue-specific extinguisher (Tse-1) locus. To this end we transfected the
same constructs used to define the liver-specific enhancer into a hepatoma
microcell hybrid line (Lem et al., 1989) which contains a small segment of human
fibroblast chromosome 17, carrying and expressing the Tse-1 locus. The enhancer
was inactive in this cell line. However, induction with cAMP was able to
overcome extinction completely, thus revealing a functional antagonism between
Tse-1 and the signal transduction pathway.

As a first step towards understanding the mechanism of extinction of enhancer
function by Tse-1, we sought to identify the specific sequences required for
liver-specific enhancer activity, for induction by cAMP and for extinction by
Tse-1. A complete set of clustered point mutants covering the enhancer was
constructed and transfected into rat hepatoma cells. Within the 80 bp minimal
enhancer fragment two short DNA sequences were found, each of which was
absolutely essential for enhancer function. Each of the two sequences was
inactive on its own, if placed in front of the heterologous TK promoter.
However, multiple copies of these sequences confered strong transcriptional
stimulation onto the TK promoter.

A multimer of the distal 26 bp sequence was responsive to cAMP and was subject
to negative regulation by Tse-1. Again the functional antagonism between Tse-1
and the cAMP-pathway was observed; cAMP induction completely reversed the

negative regulation by Tse-1. In vivo footprinting revealed characteristic changes in DMS-reactivity at this sequence element which correlated with (i) cAMP induction, (ii) the presence of the Tse-1 carrying chromosome fragment, and (iii) the relief from extinction by cAMP.

A multimer of the proximal 18 bp element behaved as a liver cell specific activator of transcription. In the natural context of the enhancer the distal cAMP- and Tse-1-responsive element must cooperate with the proximal liver-specific element to overcome the requirement for multimerisation. Artificial combination of the 26 bp- and 18 bp-sequences created an element with all the regulatory properties of the entire TAT enhancer.

Thus, the structure of the enhancer exemplifies the concept of the modular architecture of regulatory elements: a cAMP responsive module and a liver-specific module must cooperate to make up a functional unit with regulatory properties unique to the combination of both. The strict cell-type specificity of this combination is guaranteed by a double control and by the absence of redundancy: both modules are absolutely essential and both are inactive in fibroblasts. In the case of the cAMP-responsive element, which might be recognized by an ubiquitous factor, Tse-1 exerts negative control in fibroblasts.

As the balance between Tse-1 activity and cAMP induction is critical for activity of one component which is synergistically interacting with a second component, the TAT enhancer must have the properties of a sensitive switch responding to changes in the Tse-1/cAMP balance with dramatic changes in overall activity. Therefore, one attractive model would give Tse-1 a central role in prenatal repression of TAT. Activity of Tse-1 in the liver would decrease during liver development rendering the repressed TAT gene increasingly responsive to hormonal stimulation towards the end of gestation. The timed onset of TAT expression around birth would then be triggered by the strong release of gluconeogenic hormones as a consequence of neonatal hypoglycemia. In fact, TAT can be induced prematurely, days before birth by administration in utero of glucagon (acting via cAMP) (Greengard, 1970).

REFERENCES

Gluecksohn-Waelsch, S. (1979): Genetic control of morphogenetic and biochemical differentiation: lethal albino deletions in the mouse. Cell 16, 225-237.
Greengard, O. (1970): The developmental activation of enzymes in rat liver. In Mechanisms of Hormone Action, Vol. I, G. Litwack, ed. (New York: Academic Press), pp. 53-85.
Jantzen, H.M., Strähle, U., Gloss, B., Stewart, F., Schmid, W., Boshart, M., Miksicek, R., Schütz, G. (1987): Cooperativity of glucocorticoid response elements located far upstream of the tyrosine aminotransferase gene. Cell 49, 29-38.
Killary, A.M. and Fournier, R.E.K. (1984): A genetic analysis of extinction: trans-dominant loci regulate expression of liver-specific traits in hepatoma hybrid cells. Cell 38, 523-534.
Lem, J., Chin, A.C., Thayer, M.J., Leach, R.J. and Fournier, R.E.K. (1989): Coordinate regulation of two genes encoding gluconeogenic enzymes by the trans-dominant locus Tse-1. Proc. Natl. Acad. Sci. USA 85, 7302-7306.
Schmid, W., Müller, G., Schütz, G. and Gluecksohn-Waelsch, S. (1985): Deletions near the albino locus on chromosome 7 of the mouse affect the level of tyrosine aminotransferase mRNA. Proc. Natl. Acad. Sci. USA 82, 2866-2869.

Hormones and Cell Regulation. N° 14, Eds J. Nunez, J.E. Dumont. Colloque INSERM/J. Libbey Eurotext Ltd. © 1989. Vol. 198, pp. 49-55

Regulation of expression of the gene encoding aromatase cytochrome P-450

Evan R. Simpson, Sandra Graham-Lorence, C. Jo Corbin, Jill C. Merrill, Mala S. Mahendroo and Carole R. Mendelson

Cecil H. & Ida Green Center for Reproductive Biology Sciences, Departments of Obstetrics-Gynecology and Biochemistry, University of Texas Southwestern Medical Center, Dallas, Texas 75235, USA

'RODUCTION

matase is the enzyme responsible for the conversion of androgens to estrogens and comprises two ponents. The first of these is a member of the superfamily of genes known collectively as cytochrome i0 (Nebert *et al.*, 1987), namely, aromatase cytochrome P-450 (P450$_{AROM}$, P450XIX or CYP19). This ⁄me is responsible for binding of the androgen substrate and converting it to the corresponding ogen. Associated with this enzyme is a flavoprotein, NADPH-cytochrome P450 reductase, which is a quitous component of the endoplasmic reticulum of most cell types. This reductase is responsible for sferring reducing equivalents from NADPH to the cytochrome P-450$_{AROM}$ which carries out a series of e hydroxylation reactions involving 3 moles of oxygen and 3 moles of NADPH per mole of substrate ompson & Siiteri, 1974a; Thompson & Siiteri, 1974b). This results in the oxidative loss of the C$_{19}$ ılar methyl group of the androgen in the form of formic acid, and aromatization of the A-ring to give phenolic A-ring characteristic of estrogens (Akhtar *et al.*, 1982; Caspi *et al.*, 1984; Cole & Robinson, i).

sistent with its role in the biosynthesis of estrogens, this enzyme is expressed in the granulosa cells of ·ian follicles (McNatty *et al.*, 1976) where it is responsible for the estradiol produced in the follicular ie of the ovarian cycle. It is also expressed in the placenta (Fournet-Dulguerov *et al.*, 1987) where it s rise to the formation of the large quantities of estriol formed during the latter half of pregnancy. In tion, it is expressed in a number of other tissue sites including the Sertoli cell (Fritz *et al.*, 1976) and lig cells (Tsai-Morris *et al.*, 1984; Valladares & Payne, 1979) of the testis, adipose tissue (Grodin, *et al.*, ı; Edman & MacDonald, 1978), various sites of the brain including the hippocampus, medulla, and thalamus (Roselli *et al.*, 1985; Naftolin *et al.*, 1975), as well as the pre-implantation blastocyst ıgupta *et al.*, 1982). Expression of the enzyme in the brain has been implicated in the imprinting of related behavior as well the entraining of the sex-dependent pattern of GnRH secretion during adult Expression of the enzyme in adipose tissue has been implicated in at least two common malignancies omen, namely endometrial (Hemsell *et al.*, 1974; MacDonald *et al.*, 1978) and breast cancer (O'Neill ., 1988). Finally, expression of the enzyme in the blastocyst may be an implantation signal, which could ain why no deficiency of this enzyme has been recorded in contrast to all of the other steroid oxylases.

Table 1.

Issues Regarding Aromatase

1. Number of polypeptides involved in the aromatase reaction
2. Number of tissue specific forms of aromatase
3. Control of tissue specific expression
4. Mechanisms involved in the multifactorial regulation of aromatase gene expression
5. Molecular basis of clinical syndromes related to estrogen biosynthesis

Table 1 lists a number of interesting questions related to this enzyme. In order to address these issues we have isolated and characterized cDNA inserts complementary to mRNA encoding cytochrome P-450$_{AROM}$. These inserts have been expressed in order to characterize the nature of the reaction catalyzed by the single protein expressed by the cDNAs. Furthermore, these cDNAs have been used in turn to screen human genomic libraries in order to isolate and characterize the gene encoding cytochrome P-450$_{AROM}$.

EXPRESSION OF cDNAs ENCODING AROMATASE CYTOCHROME P-450.

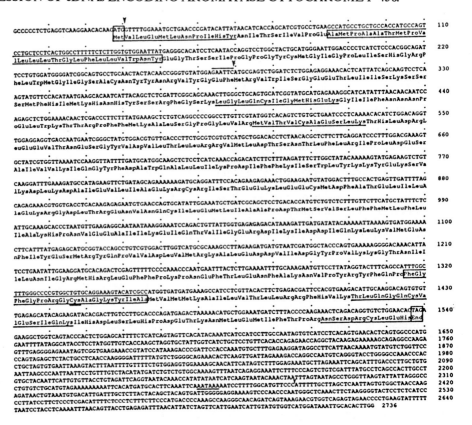

Fig. 1　Sequence of full-length cDNA encoding human cytochrome P-450$_{AROM}$. The beginning and end of the open reading frame are indicated by *boxes*. The start of a previously characterized 2.5 kb cDNA clone is indicated by the *second arrow*, and just upstream from this is indicated an internal *Eco*RI restriction site. Indicated by the *boxed areas* are the putative membrane spanning domain and heme-binding region. Within the 3'-untranslated region an internal polyadenylation signal is indicated, and 20 base pairs downstream, a *third arrow* indicates the start of the poly(A$^+$) tail of another cDNA clone which otherwise appears identical to this one

tially, a human placental λgt11 cDNA library was screened using polyclonal and monoclonal antibodies prepared against human cytochrome P-450$_{AROM}$. A partial cDNA insert was isolated from this library and s used to rescreen a λgt10 placental library and also a primer-extended library (Evans *et al.*, 1986; npson *et al.*, 1987; Corbin *et al.*, 1988). On the basis of these studies a full-length cDNA insert was lated and characterized as shown in Figure 1. This insert contains an open reading frame characteristic a microsomal cytochrome P-450, in that it contains at the N-terminal region a hydrophobic sequence of ino acids suggestive of a membrane-spanning domain. Furthermore, at the carboxy-terminal end there region of high homology with other cytochrome P-450 species which is believed to be the heme-binding ion of these enzymes, and contains at its center a histidine residue which is believed to be the fifth rdinating ligand of the heme iron. In order to express this cDNA, it was inserted into a modified MV expression vector and used to transfect COS-1 monkey kidney tumor cells using the DEAE-tran method. The kinetic data obtained are summarized in Table 2 (Corbin *et al.*, 1988).

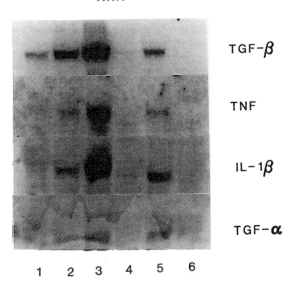

Human Adipose Stromal Cell
RNA

						TGF-β
						TNF
						IL-1β
						TGF-α
1	2	3	4	5	6	

. 2   Effects of various growth factors on the levels of mRNA encoding cytochrome P-450$_{AROM}$ as determined by Northern analysis. Lane 1: no additions; lane 2: (Bu)$_2$cAMP; lane 3: (Bu)$_2$cAMP + PDA; lane 4: (Bu)$_2$cAMP + growth factor; lane 5: (Bu)$_2$cAMP + PDA + growth factor; lane 6: growth factor alone.

Table 2.

Kinetic Properties of Cytochrome P-450$_{AROM}$ Expressed in COS1 Cells

Substrate	K_m (nM)	V_{max} (pmol·h^{-1}·mg^{-1} pr
[1β-^{3}H]Androstenedione	50 ± 18[+]	102 ± 59[+]
[1,2-^{3}H]Testosterone	55 ± 7[+]	148 ± 58[+]
[1β-^{3}H]16α-Hydroxyandrostenedione	99[‡]	11[‡]

[+] Mean ± S.E.M. of 3 determinations
[‡] Mean of 2 determinations

It can be seen that the expressed cytochrome P-450$_{AROM}$ protein was capable of aromatizing all th substrates, namely androstenedione, testosterone, and 16α-hydroxyandrostenedione, to the correspond products, namely, estrone, estradiol, and 16α-hydroxyestrone. Moreover, the K_m and V_{max} values obtain are within the range of those previously ascribed to the purified human placental P-450$_{AROM}$ prote (Kellis & Vickery, 1987). Based on these results, it is apparent that a single P-450$_{AROM}$ species c metabolize the three major types of androgen substrate encountered in the human. And moreover, ea of these substrates can be converted to the corresponding estrogen. Thus, it is apparent that unnecessary to postulate the existence of more than one aromatase enzyme within the human organism.

This cDNA has also been used in Northern analysis to study the regulation of expression of cytochrome 450$_{AROM}$ in human ovarian granulosa cells (Steinkampf et al., 1987; Steinkampf et al., 1988), as well as human adipose stromal cells (Simpson et al., 1989). In each of these cell types the expression of t P450$_{AROM}$ mRNA is enhanced by cyclic AMP analogs. However, in other aspects the regulation is qu different. For example, in adipose stromal cells, phorbol esters markedly potentiate the action of dibuty cAMP to increase the expression of this enzyme (Mendelson et al., 1986), whereas in ovarian granulc cells phorbol esters are inhibitory. Moreover, in adipose stromal cells, a number of growth factors inhi the expression of P450$_{AROM}$ mRNA in the presence of dibutyryl cAMP or of dibutyryl cAMP plus phorl esters. These include EGF, PDGF, FGF, TGF-β, TGF-α, IL-1β, and TNF (Simpson et al., 198 Mendelson et al., 1986). The results of some of these studies are summarized in Figure 2. Thus, it apparent that cytochrome P-450$_{AROM}$ is subject not only to tissue-specific regulation but to compl multifactorial regulation by a number of factors, and that the regulation of expression differs in the vario cell types in which it is expressed.

CHARACTERIZATION OF THE GENE ENCODING HUMAN AROMATASE CYTOCHROME P-450.

In order to find a basis for understanding the regulation of expression of P-450$_{AROM}$, it was clea necessary to isolate and characterize the gene encoding this enzyme. Accordingly, human genom libraries in EMBL-3 and Charon-4A were screened using the cDNA inserts encoding P-450$_{AROM}$. On th basis of this, four genomic clones were characterized which spanned the entire gene as shown in Figure The gene is greater than 52 kb long and contains 10 exons. The first of these is in the 5'-untranslat region of the gene and is separated from the start of translation by an intron that is at least 19 kb long, b since these clones have not been overlapped, the exact size of this intron is unclear. In common with oth cytochrome P-450 species, the heme-binding region is encoded by the last exon which also encodes th entire 3'-untranslated region. This region contains two putative polyadenylation signals accounting for th two mRNA species which are observed, one of 3.4 kb and one of 2.9 kb. Comparison of the location of th exon-intron junctions with those of human 21-hydroxylase P-450 and 17α-hydroxylase P-450, the oth microsomal steroidogenic P-450s, reveals that whereas there is a remarkable coincidence in the locatio of these boundaries in the case of the latter two enzymes, the localization of these boundaries aromatase cytochrome P-450 differs markedly, indicating that cytochrome P-450$_{AROM}$ likely diverg before the appearance of 21-hydroxylase and 17α-hydroxylase cytochrome P-450s. The sequence of the 5'-untranslated region has been determined, and primer extension analysis revealed a start of transcription some 23 base pairs downstream from a putative TATA box, as well as the existence of three possible CAT boxes. Other putative regulatory sequences in this region include a sequence with reasonable homology to the CRE consensus sequence at position -211, two putative GRE sequences, one at position -358 and one at position +346 in the first intron, which actually has a perfect hexamer canonical GRE sequence. There is also a sequence resembling an AP-1 site within the 5'-untranslated region at -54 bp. Deletion mutations containing these sequences are being inserted upstream of suitable reporter genes in order to study the effect of these sequences on expression of reporter genes, thus enabling us to dissect the regions of the gene responsible for the complex regulation of expression of this enzyme.

The genes for a number of steroidogenic cytochromes P-450, including 21-hydroxylase cytochrome P-450, 17α-hydroxylase cytochrome P-450, and cholesterol side-chain cleavage cytochrome P-450 have been characterized in a number of laboratories (Morohashi et al., 1987; Picado-Leonard & DuPont, 1986; White et al., 1986). The polypeptides encoded by these genes, as well as cytochrome P-450$_{AROM}$, have considerable sequence homology leading to the speculation that they have evolved from a common ancestral gene. However, the genes differ markedly in size, ranging from ≈3 kb for P-450$_{C21}$ (White et al., 1986), to ≈7 kb for P-450$_{17α}$ (Picado-Leonard & DuPont, 1986), to >20 kb for P450$_{scc}$ (Morohashi et al., 1987) and >52 kb for aromatase (Means et al., unpublished observations). It is of interest that all of these genes, which encode polypeptides of similar molecular weight, are comprised of 8-10 exons of roughly similar size, suggesting a subdivision of functional domains; however, the sizes of the intervening sequences vary widely.

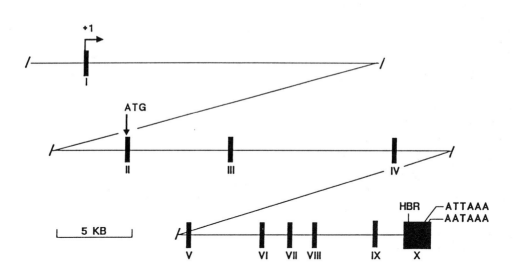

Fig. 3   Schematic of the gene encoding human cytochrome P-450$_{AROM}$. Restriction sites for Sal I (S), Hind III (H) and EcoRI (E) are indicated, as are the ten exons (I-X). The gene spans four clones as indicated, the first containing an untranslated exon. The 2nd and 3rd clones overlap, whereas the others do not.

CONCLUSIONS

Human cytochrome P-450$_{AROM}$ is encoded by a single copy gene of at least 52 kb in length, which is transcribed into two mRNA species that differ in the lengths of their 3'-untranslated regions. These mRNA species encode a single polypeptide which has the capacity to catalyze all of the enzymatic steps involved in the aromatization of C_{19}-steroids to estrogens. Our findings also are indicative that a single species of cytochrome P-450$_{AROM}$ is capable of aromatizing androstenedione, testosterone, and 16α hydroxyandrostenedione, resulting in the formation of estrone, estradiol-17β, and estriol, respectively, as the major products. Thus, it is likely that only one enzyme is responsible for the aromatization of C_{19} steroids in humans. Finally, hormonally-induced alterations in aromatase activity of human ovarian granulosa cells are associated with comparable changes in the levels of P-450$_{AROM}$ mRNA. Studies are in progress to define the molecular mechanisms whereby stimulatory and inhibitory factors regulate P 450$_{AROM}$ gene expression in estrogen-producing cells.

ACKNOWLEDGEMENTS

This work was supported by USPHS grants AM31206 and AG08174. S.G.L. was supported, in part, by USPHS training grant 5-T32-HD07190.

REFERENCES

Akhtar, M., Calder, M.R., Corina, D.L. & Wright, J.N. (1982): Mechanistic studies on C-19 demethylation in oestrogen biosynthesis. *Biochem. J.* 201, 569-580.

Caspi, E., Wicha, J., Arunachalam, T., Nelson, P. & Spiteller, G. (1984): Estrogen biosynthesis Concerning the obligatory intermediacy of 2β-hydroxy-10β-formylandrost-4-ene-3,17-dione. *J. Am Chem. Soc.* 106, 7282-7283.

Cole, P.A. & Robinson, C.H. (1988): A peroxide model reaction for placental aromatase. *J. Am. Chem Soc.* 110, 1284-1285.

Corbin, C.J., Graham-Lorence, S., McPhaul, M., Mason, J.I., Mendelson, C.R. & Simpson, E.R. (1988) Isolation of a full-length cDNA insert encoding human aromatase system cytochrome P-450 and its expression in nonsteroidogenic cells. *Proc. Natl. Acad. Sci. USA* 85, 8948-8952.

Edman, C.D. & MacDonald, P.C. (1978): Effect of obesity on conversion of plasma androstenedione to estrone in ovulatory and anovulatory young women. *Am. J. Obstet. Gynecol.* 130, 456-461.

Evans, C.T., Ledesma, D.B., Schulz, T.Z., Simpson, E.R. & Mendelson, C.R. (1986): Isolation and characterization of a complementary cDNA specific for human aromatase cytochrome P-450. *Proc. Natl. Acad. Sci. USA* 83, 6387-6391.

Fournet-Dulguerov, N., MacLusky, N.J., Leranth, C.Z., Todd, R., Mendelson, C.R., Simpson, E.R. & Naftolin, F. (1987): Immunological localization of aromatase cytochrome P-450 and estradiol dehydrogenase in the syncytiotrophoblast of the human placenta. *J. Clin. Endocrinol. Metab.* 65, 757-764.

Fritz, I.B., Griswold, M.D., Louis, B.F. & Dorrington, J.H. (1976): Similarity of responses of cultured Sertoli cells to cholera toxin and FSH. *Mol. Cell. Endocrinol.* 5, 289-294.

Grodin, J.M., Siiteri, P.K. & MacDonald, P.C. (1973): Source of estrogen production in the postmenopausal women. *J. Clin. Endocrinol. Metab.* 36, 207-214.

Hemsell, D.L., Grodin, J.M., Breuner, P.F., Siiteri, P.K. & MacDonald, P.C. (1974): Plasma precursors of estrogen II correlation of the extent of conversion of plasma androstenedione to estrone with age. *J. Clin. Endocrinol. Metab.* 38, 476-479.

Kellis, J.T. & Vickery, L.E. (1987): Purification and characterization of human placental aromatase cytochrome P-450. *J. Biol. Chem.* 262, 4413-4420.

MacDonald, P.C., Edman, C.D., Hemsell, D.L., Porter, J.C. & Siiteri, P.K. (1978): Effect of obesity on conversion of plasma androstenedione to estrone in postmenopausal women with and without endometrial cancer. *Am. J. Obstet. Gynecol.* 130, 448-455.

McNatty, K.P., Baird, D.T., Bolton, A., Chambers, P., Corker, C.S. & MacLean, H. (1976): Concentrations of oestrogens and androgens in human ovarian venous plasma and follicular fluid throughout the menstrual cycle. *J. Endocrinol.* 71, 77-85.

Mendelson, C.R., Corbin, C.J., Smith, M.E., Smith, J. & Simpson, E.R. (1986): Growth factors suppress and phorbol esters potentiate the action of dibutyryl cyclic AMP to stimulate aromatase activity of human adipose stromal cells. *Endocrinology* 118, 968-973.

Morohashi, K, Sagawa, K., Omura, T. & Fujii-Kuriyama, Y. (1987): Gene structure of human cytochrome P450(Scc), cholesterol desmolase. *J. Biochem.* 101, 879-887.

aftolin, F., Ryan, K.J., Davies, I.J., Reddy, V.V., Flores, F., Petro, Z., Kuhn, M., White, R.J., Takosha, Y. & Wolin, L. (1975): The formation of estrogen by central neuroendocrine tissues. *Recent Prog. Horm. Res.* 31, 295-319.

ebert, D.W., Adesnik, M., Coon, M.J., Estabrook, R.W., Gonzalez, F.J., Guengerich, F.P., Gunsalus, I.C., Johnson, E.F., Kemper, B., Levin, W., Philips, I.R., Sato, R. & Waterman, M.R. (1987): The P-450 gene superfamily: recommended nomenclature. *DNA* 6, 1-11.

Neill, J.S., Elton, R.A. & Miller, W.A. (1988): Aromatase activity in adipose tissue from breast quandrants: a link with tumor site. *Brit. Med. J.* 296, 741-743.

cado-Leonard, J. & Miller, W.L. (1987): Cloning and sequence of the human gene for P-450$_{C17}$ (steroid 17α-hydroxylase/17,20 lyase): Similarily with the gene for P-450$_{C21}$. *DNA* 6, 439-448.

oselli, C.E., Horton, L.E. & Resko, J.A. (1985): Distribution and regulation of aromatase activity in the rat hypothalamus and limbic systems. *Endocrinology* 117, 2471-2477.

ngupta, J., Roy, S.K. & Manchada, S.K. (1982): Effect of an estrogen inhibitor, 1,4,6-androstatriene-3,17-dione, on mouse embryo development *in vitro*. *J. Reprod. Fertil.* 66, 63-65.

npson, E.R., Evans, C.T., Corbin, C.J., Powell, F.E., Ledesma, D.B. & Mendelson, C.R. (1987): Sequencing of cDNA inserts encoding aromatase cytochrome P-450 (P-450$_{AROM}$). *Mol. Cell. Endocrinol.* 52, 267-272.

npson, E.R., Merrill, J.C., Hollub, A.J., Graham-Lorence, S. & Mendelson, C.R. (1989): Regulation of estrogen biosynthesis by human adipose tissue. *Endo. Rev.* 10, 136-148.

einkampf, M.P., Mendelson, C.R. & Simpson, E.R. (1987): Regulation by FSH of the synthesis of aromatase cytochrome P-450 (P-450$_{AROM}$) in human granulosa cells. *Mol. Endocrinol.* 1, 465-471.

einkampf, M.P., Mendelson, C.R. & Simpson, E.R. (1988): Effects of epidermal growth factor and insulin-like growth factor-I on the levels of mRNA encoding aromatase cytochrome P-450 in human ovarian granulosa cells. *Mol. Cell. Endocrinol.* 59, 93-99.

ompson, Jr., E.A. & Siiteri, P.K. (1974a): Utilization of oxygen and reduced nicotinamide adenine dinucleotide phosphate by human placental microsomes during aromatization of androstenedione. *J. Biol. Chem.* 249, 5364-5372.

ompson, Jr., E.A. & Siiteri, P.K. (1974b): The involvement of human placental microsomal cytochrome P-450 in aromatization. *J. Biol. Chem.* 249, 5373-5380.

ai-Morris, C.H., Aquilano, D.R. & Dufau, M.L. (1984): Gonadotropic regulation of aromatase activity in the adult rat testis. *Ann. NY Acad. Sci.* 43, 666-669.

illadares, L.E. & Payne, A.H. (1979): Induction of testicular aromatization by luteinizing hormone in mature rats. *Endocrinology* 105, 431-436.

hite, P.C., New, M.I. & DuPont, B. (1986): Structure of human steroid 21-hydroxylase genes. *Proc. Natl. Acad. Sci. USA* 83, 511-515.

Hormones and Cell Regulation. N° 14, Eds J. Nunez, J.E. Dumont. Colloque INSERM/J. Libbey Eurotext Ltd. © 1989. Vol. 198, pp. 57-62

AP1 and PEA3 are nuclear targets for transcription activation by non-nuclear oncogenes

P. Flores, A. Gutman, J.L. Imler, A. Lloyd, J. Schneikert, C. Wasylyk and B. Wasylyk*

Laboratoire de Génétique Moléculaire des Eucaryotes du CNRS, Unité 184 de Biologie Moléculaire et de Génie Génétique de l'INSERM, Institut de Chimie Biologique, Faculté de Médecine, 11 rue Humann 67085 Strasbourg Cédex, France

* Corresponding author

We have found that the activity of the transcription factor PEA3 is regulated by the expression of non-nuclear oncogenes. This factor, although it is distinct from PEA1 (AP1), is activated by the same oncogenes (v-src, polyoma (Py) middle T, c-Ha-ras, v-mos, v-raf), by TPA and by serum components. However, in contrast to PEA1, c-fos does not appear to be necessary for activation of PEA3, suggesting that PEA3 is a fos-independent target for regulation of transcription by non-nuclear oncogenes.

INTRODUCTION

In order to understand how many different oncogenes can transform cells, it is important to identify common regulatory events. Recent studies have linked the effects of non-nuclear oncogenes to the activity of the transcription factor AP1 or PEA1 (reviewed in Imler & Wasylyk, 1989 ; Herrlich & Ponta, 1989). AP1 is a composite factor, consisting of heterodimers between c-fos and c-jun gene-family members (Curran & Franza, 1988). The canonical members of these families are themselves proto-oncogenes (Vogt & Tjian, 1988) suggesting than an important event in cell transformation by non-nuclear oncogenes could be altered AP1 activity. However, to understand the diverse effects that non-nuclear oncogenes can have on gene expression, it is important to identify other nuclear targets. We have shown that the same oncogenes that alter PEA1 (AP1) activity also regulate the activity of PEA3. PEA1 and PEA3 are distinct factors, which interact with different motifs of the α domain of the Py enhancer (Martin et al., 1988 ; see below). The potential role of PEA3 in the regulation of cellular gene transcription is discussed.

PEA3, a transcription factor distinct from PEA1 (AP1) which has a similar pattern of induction by non-nuclear oncogenes, TPA and serum

There are three characterised, distinct transcription factors which bind to the α domain of the Py-enhancer, PEA1, PEA2 and PEA3 (Piette and Yaniv, 1987 ; Martin et al., 1988 ; Imler et al., 1988, this work). Two of these, PEA1 and PEA3, share the property of being inducible by oncogene expression, serum, and TPA (unlike PEA2, Wasylyk et al., 1988b ; Satake et al., 1988). The evidence that PEA3 and PEA1 are different factors is : 1) they both binds only to their own, distinct motif in vitro, 2) PEA1 expressed in vivo does not activate the PEA3 motif, even though this motif has an inducible activity, 3) PEA1 and PEA3 have distinct patterns of induction by serum in vitro, 4) they have different behaviours towards fos expression, both in vivo and in vitro. Despite these difference they share the following properties : 1) their activity is inducible in vivo by non-nuclear oncogenes (v-src, Py-mt, Ha-ras, v-mos, v-raf), serum and TPA, 2) their DNA binding properties are altered by serum ingredients, oncogene expression and cell-transformation, (see also Piette et al., 1988 for PEA1) 3) their activity in vivo is not induced by the oncogenes SV40-LT, Py-LT, myc, EIA, BPV E2 and E5. What is the significance of these common properties ?

There is some evidence that the non-nuclear oncogenes may be linked in the process of signal transduction from the exterior of the cell to the nucleus, in the order serum → src + Py-mt → ras + protein kinase C → mos → raf → jun + fos (for Discussions, see Schonthal et al., 1988 ; Wasylyk et al., 1988a ; Herrlich and Ponta, 1989 ; Imler and Wasylyk, 1989). Our present observations are consistent with the existence of such a pathway, since a second distinct factor is activated by the same oncogenes. They also predict that the events on this pathway that regulate PEA3 activity are downstream from raf, and independent of c-fos and c-jun. Several lines of evidence suggest that PEA3 activity is independent from that of fos or jun 1) fos or jun expression does not affect PEA3-motif activity in vivo, 2) fos expression does not alter PEA3 specific DNA-binding activity in vitro, 3) the same c-fos anti-sense RNA, which inhibits oncogene activation of the collagenase TRE (Schönthal et al., 1988) does not appear to block oncogene induction of PEA3 activity (P. Flores, in preparation).

These results suggest that PEA3 is a primary target for signal transduction, which should therefore respond rapidly to extra-cellular signals. How can this prediction be reconciled with the slow induction in vitro of PEA3 DNA binding activity relative to PEA1. We have recently shown that PEA3 activity is maximally induced at the latest 1h after serum or TPA stimulation of LMTK⁻ cells, and that this activation is not prevented by blocking protein synthesis with cycloheximide (P. Flores, in preparation, see also Wasylyk et al., 1988b). These results suggest that there are two aspects to the control of PEA3 activity, a rapid post-translational mechanism, and a slower accumulation of protein (DNA-binding activity). Similar, bi-modal mechanisms of activation appear to be shared by AP1 (PEA1, Brenner et al., 1989 ; Angel et al., 1988b ; Schonthal et al., 1988) and SRF (Norman et al., 1988 ; Prywes et al., 1988), and may account for short and long term responses to cellular signals.

Co-operation between different factors in the response to oncogene induction

The emerging evidence for multiple targets in the nucleus for growth factor/oncogene activation leads to the question how these signals are integrated into coordinate regulation during the cell cycle. Growth factors, serum and oncogenes elicit distinct patterns of induction of c-jun and jun-B (Pertovaara et al., 1989 ; Quantin and Breathnach, 1988 ; Ryseck et al., 1988 ; Lamph et al., 1988 ; Ryder and Nathans, 1988 ; Ryder et al., 1988) whereas the levels of the third known member of the gene family, jun-D, remains constant (Hirai et al., 1989 ; Ryder et al., 1989). At least three members of the fos gene family are induced with different kinetics during the cell-cycle (Cohen and Curran, 1988 ; Zerial et al., 1989 ; Gentz et al., 1989). Several members of the fos and jun gene families can form heterodimers (see for example Cohen et al., 1989 ; Neuberg et al., Gentz et al., 1989 ; Turner and Tjian, 1989 ; Zerial et al., 1989) suggesting that at different times in the cell-cycle, different heterodimers can form. Presumably, the specificity for activation of transcription lies in the sequences that these composite transcription factors can bind to (see Quinn et al., 1989, for example), and also in the possible interacions they may have with other transcription factors. The α domain of the Py-enhancer may provide a useful model in understanding some aspects of these interactions.

We found by co-transfection experiments that oncogene induction of PEA1-motif activity could be complemented by c-fos, but not not c-jun or jun-B. These results agree with known properties of c-jun and c-fos induction. The c-jun gene promoter is positively regulated by its own gene product, and this is thought to account for the prolonged induction of c-jun gene transcription relative to c-fos in certain conditions (Brenner et al., 1989). Similar differences in kinetics would readily account for the observation that for both src, a good inducer of PEA1, or ras, a poorer inducer of PEA1, the limiting component is fos. However, the mechanism may be more complex than this, and other unknown elements may have to be taken into account, including the effects of oncogenes on the amount and specific activity of other members of the fos (eg. fra-1, Cohen and Curran, 1988 ; fos B, Zerial et al., 1989) and jun (jun-D, Hirai et al., 1989 ; Ryder et al., 1989) gene families, and their relative affinities for the particular PEA1 motif in the Py α domain.

Some of our results suggest that there could be cooperative interactions between some component(s) of PEA1 and PEA3. 1) The PEA3 motif alone is not as inducible as the α domain oligonucleotides PB or M5, even though this sequence is sufficient for efficient binding of PEA3. 2). Several different PEA1-like motifs, in the absence of a PEA3 motif, are less inducible by oncogene expression than the Py α domain (our unpublished results). Further studies are required to identify and characterise interacting components on the α domain of Py enhancer.

Potential role of PEA3 in cellular and viral gene transcription

5'-CAGGAAGTGAC-3'
Human transferrin receptor	(HSTR5,35)
Human factor IX	(HSFIXG,2770)
Rat fibrinogen gamma chain	(RNFIBG1,419)
Human Adenovirus 5 EIA enhancer	(ADEE1AED,4)
Human Spumaretrovirus LTR	(RESPULTR,1271)
Polyomavirus enhancer	(POLLAT,164)

5'-CAGGAAGTG-3'
Human interleukin 2	(HSIL05,938)
Human 2-5A synthetase	(HS25ASYP,468)
Human interferon inducible IFI-54K	(HSINIFI,113)
Mouse nerve growth factor α-subunit	(MMNGFA1,76)
Rat fibrinogen alpha chain	(RNFBAG,1540)
Rat metallothionein-2	(RNMT12C,338)
Rat thyroglobulin	(RNTHYRP,181)
Rat U2 small nuclear RNA	(RNUG2A,333)
Chicken δ-2 crystallin	(GGCRY,324)
Drosophila alcohol dehydrogenase	(DOADHG,463)
Yeast LTE1	(SCLTE1,110)
Yeast MRS3	(SCMRS3,250)
EBV early cytoplasmic antigen	(EBV,53502)

5'-CAGGATGT-3'
Human/mouse c-fos	(MMCFOS,236)

5'-GAGGATGT-3'
Human/rabbit collagenase	(MSCN2A,436)

5'-CAGGAAGCATTTCCTG-3'
Rat/rabbit stromelysin	(RNTRAN,900)

Fig. 1. Promoters with sequence homology to the PEA3 motif. The EMBL nucleotide sequence data bank was searched for perfect homologies to either an 11 bp or 9 bp sequence from around the PEA3 motif of the Py enhancer α domain. Only homologies within sequences upstream from RNA startsites are shown. In addition, several closely related sequences in the c-fos, collagenase and stromelysin-transin promoters are shown. The sequence name in the data-bank, and the position of the first C are in parentheses.

We can expect that the Py virus has adopted cellular regulatory mechanism for the control of its enhancer. As a preliminary approach to understanding the role of PEA3 in the regulation of cellular and viral promoters, we have searched through the EMBL data bank for regions upstream from mRNA startsites with complete sequence homology to either 11 bp or 9 bp sequences from around the PEA3 motif (Fig. 1). We also searched for related sequences, but only in promoters which are known to be inducible by oncogene expression (Fig. 1). There is evidence that some of these homologies could be functionally significant.

Some of the promoters with PEA3 motifs can be grouped according to the types of inducers which activate their transcription : 1) acute phase response (α and γ fibrinogen ; Fowles et al., 1984) 2) γ interferon (2-5A synthetase and IFI-54 K ; Wathelet et al., 1988) 3) mitogens and oncogenes (transferrin receptor, Ad EIA enhancer, interleukin-2, metallothionein-2, EBV early cytoplasmic, collagenase, stromolysin, c-fos). The role of the PEA3 motif in the first two responses is unknown, but there is some evidence for a role in mediating the effect of mitogens and oncogenes on the other promoters. The transferrin receptor promoter is activated by mitogens, and the PEA3 like sequence is located in the minimum promoter element required for both transcription activity and specific binding of proteins in extracts (Miskimins et al., 1986). The Ad EIA enhancer is repressed by EIA and activated by E1B (Yoshida et al., 1987), which is reminiscent of the opposing effect of EIA and non-nuclear oncogenes (which share transforming properties with E1B) on PEA3 activity. Activation of the interleukin 2 promoter with TPA and phytohemagglutinin in T cells leads to changes in the pattern of binding of proteins to several parts of the promoter, one of which encompasses the PEA3 motif (B' site, Nabel et al., 1988). The EBV early cytoplasmic antigen promoter (BHRF1) is inducible by TPA, and subsequent transcription of BHRF1 is associated with entry into the lytic cycle in B cells (Hardwick et al., 1988). We have observed that PEA3 activity is low in myeloma cells, and is activated by TPA and oncogene expression (our unpublished results) showing that the PEA3 motif can be a responsive element in B cells. The BHRF1 promoter also has a PEA1/AP1 like motif, and is activated by the Z trans-activator which has sequence similarity with c-fos, c-jun and GN-4 (Farrell et al., 1989). AP1/PEA1 motifs are associated with PEA3 motifs in the collagenase, stromelysin (transin) and c-fos promoters, suggesting that the association could have functional significance. The collagenase PEA3-like motif specifically binds proteins present in cell-extracts (Angel et al., 1987a), and it has been noted that there are unidentified elements in this promoter besides the TRE (AP1-motif) which mediated TPA induction of promoter activity (Angel et al., 1987a). The stromelysin PEA3 like motif is present as a palindrome (see Fig. 1), in a region of the promoter which is completely conserved between rabbits and rats (Frish and Ruley, 1987). The PEA3 like motif in the c-fos promoter is required for the response of the c-fos promoter to serum, and is the binding site for p62, which participates in the formation of a ternary complex over the serum response element (Shaw et al., 1989). The enticing possibility is that p62 is related to PEA3, and that this factor(s) is involved in early events in signal transduction leading to induction of c-fos transcription.

60

REFERENCES

Angel, P., Imagawa, M., Chiu, R., Stein, B., Imbra, R.J., Rahmsdorf, H.J., Jonat, C., Herrlich, P. and Karin, M. (1987a) Cell 49, 729-739.

Angel, P., Baumann, I., Stein, B., Delius, H., Rahmsdorf, H.J. and Herrlich, P. (1987b) Mol. Cell. Biol. 7, 2256-2266.

Angel, P., Allegretto, E.A., Okino, S.T., Hattori, K., Boyle, W.J., Hunter, T. and Karin, M. (1988a) Nature 332, 166-171.

Angel, P., Hattori, K., Smeal, T. and Karin, M. (1988b) Cell 55, 875-885.

Bartel, D.P., Sheng, M., Lau, L.F. and Greenberg, M.E. (1989) Genes and Development 3, 304-313.

Brenner, D.A., O'Hara, M., Angel, P., Chojkier, M. and Karin, M. (1989) Nature 337, 661-663.

Cohen, D.R. and Curran, T. (1988) Mol. Cell. Biol. 8, 2063-2069.

Cohen, D.R., Ferreira, P.C.P., Gentz, R., Franza Jr., B.R. and Curran, T. (1989) Genes and Development 3, 173-184.

Curran, T. and Franza Jr., B.R. (1988) Cell 55, 395-397.

Farrell, P.J., Rowe, D.T., Rooney, C.M. and Kouzarides, T. (1989) EMBO J. 8, 127-132.

Fowlkes, D.M., Mullis, N.T., Comeau, C.M. and Crabtree, G.R. (1984) Proc. Natl. Acad. Sci. USA 81, 2313-2316.

Frisch, S.M. and Ruley, H.E. (1987) J. Biol. Chem. 262, 16300-16304.

Gentz, R., Rauscher III, F.J., Abate, C. and Curran T. (1989) Science 243, 1695-1699.

Hardwick, J.M., Lieberman, P.M. and Hayward, S.D. (1988) J. Virology 62, 2274-2284.

Herrlich, P. and Ponta, H. (1989) Trends in Genetics, in press.

Hirai, S.I., Ryseck, R.P., Mechta, F., Bravo, R., and Yaniv, M. (1989) EMBO J., in press.

Imler, J.L., Schatz, C., Wasylyk, C., Chatton, B. and Wasylyk, B. (1988) Nature 332, 275-278.

Imler, J.L. and Wasylyk, B. (1989) In "Progress in Growth Factor Research", J.K. Heath (ed.), Pergamon Press, in press.

Lamph, W.W., Wamsley, P., Sassone-Corsi, P. and Verma, I.M. (1988) Nature 334, 629-631.

Martin, M.E., Piette, J., Yaniv, M., Tang, W.J. and Folk, W.R. (1988) Proc. Natl. Acad. Sci. USA 85, 5839-5843.

Miskimins, W.K., McClelland, A., Roberts, M.P. and Ruddle, F.H. (1986) J. Cell Biol. 103, 1781-1788.

Nabel, G.J., Gorka, C. and Baltimore, D. (1988) Proc. Natl. Acad. Sci. USA 85, 2934-2938.

Neuberg, M., Schuermann, M., Hunter, J.B. and Müller, R. (1989) Nature 338, 589-590.

Norman, C., Runswick, M., Pollock, R. and Treisman, R. (1988) Cell 55, 989-1003.

Pertovaara, L., Sistonen, L., Bos, T.J., Vogt, P.K., Keski-Oja, J. and Alitalo, K. (1989) Mol. Cell. Biol. 9, 1255-1262.

Piette, J. and Yaniv, M. (1987) EMBO J. 6, 1331-1337.

Piette, J., Hirai, S.I. and Yaniv, M. (1988) Proc. Natl. Acad. Sci. USA 85, 3401-3405.

Prywes, R., Dutta, A., Cromlish, J.A. and Roeder, R.G. (1988) Proc. Natl. Acad. Sci. USA 85, 7206-7210.

Quantin, B. and Breathnach, R. (1988) Nature 334, 538-539.

Quinn, J.P., Takimoto, M., Iadarola, M., Holbrook, N. and Levens, D. (1989) J. Virology 63, 1737-1742.

Ryder, K. and Nathans, D. (1988) Proc. Natl. Acad. Sci. USA 85, 8464-8467.

Ryder, K., Lau, L.F. and Nathans, D. (1988) Proc. Natl. Acad. Sci. USA 85, 1487-1491.
Ryder, K., Lanahan, A., Perez-Albuerne, E. and Nathans, D. (1989) Proc. Natl. Acad. Sci. USA 86, 1500-1503.
Ryseck, R.P., Hirai, S.I., Yaniv, M. and Bravo, R. (1988) Nature 334, 535-537.
Satake, M., Ibaraki, T. and Ito, Y. (1988) Gene 3, 69-78.
Schönthal, A., Herrlich, P., Rahmsdorf, H.J. and Ponta, H. (1988) Cell 54, 325-334.
Shaw, P.E., Schröter, H. and Nordheim, A. (1989) Cell 56, 563-572.
Sistonen, L., Höltta, E., Makela, T.P., Keski-Oja, J. and Alitalo, K. (1989) EMBO J. 8, 815-122.
Turner, R. and Tjian, R. (1989) Science 243, 1689-1694.
Vogt, P.K. and Tjian, R. (1988) Oncogene 3, 3-7.
Wasylyk, C., Imler, J.L. and Wasylyk, B. (1988a) EMBO J. 7, 2475-2483.
Wasylyk, B., Imler, J.L., Chatton, B., Schatz, C. and Wasylyk, C. (1988b) Proc. Natl. Acad. Sci. USA 85, 7952-7956.
Wathelet, M.G., Clauss, I.M., Content, J. and Huez, G.A. (1988) Eur. J. Biochem. 174, 323-329.
Yoshida, K.L., Venkatesh, L., Kuppuswamy, M. and Chinnadurai, G. (1987) Genes and Dev. 1, 645-658.
Yu, S.F., von Rüden, T., Kantoff, P.W., Garber, C., Seiberg, M., Rüther, U., Anderson, W.F., Wagner, E.F. and Gilboa, E. (1986) Proc. Natl. Acad. Sci. USA 83, 3194-3198.
Zerial, M., Toshi, L., Ryseck, R.P., Schuermann, M., Müller, R. and Bravo, R. (1989) EMBO J. 8, 805-813.

Nous avons montré que l'activité transcriptionnelle des facteurs PEA1 et PEA3 est régulée par l'expression de certains oncogènes transformants : tels que v-src, moyen T de polyome, cHa-ras, v-mos, v-raf, ainsi que par le TPA et des composants du sérum. Malgrés ces points communs, ces facteurs sont différents. Contrairement à PEA1, PEA3 ne nécessite pas c-fos pour son activation.

Growth factors

Facteurs de croissance

Hormones and Cell Regulation. N° 14, Eds J. Nunez, J.E. Dumont. Colloque INSERM/J. Libbey Eurotext Ltd. © 1989. Vol. 198, pp. 65-70

The epidermal growth factor receptor and its role in cell transformation

Thierry J. Velu*, Patrick Martin*, William C. Vass*, Kristian Helin**, Armin Ritzhaupt*, Laura Beguinot**, John T. Schiller* and Douglas R. Lowy*.

*Laboratory of Cellular Oncology, National Cancer Institute, NIH, Bldg 37 Room 1B26, Bethesda, Maryland-20892, USA and **University Institute of Microbiology, 1353 Copenhagen K, Denmark*

INTRODUCTION

Oncogenes (*onc*), as a group, are genes that contribute directly to tumorigenesis. Cellular oncogenes (c-*onc*), or proto-oncogenes, are cellular genes which can give rise to oncogenes when their sequences are altered or when their expression is modified (Bishop, 1987). Their conservation in the evolution and their role in cell transformation suggest that c-*onc* play key roles in the control of normal cell growth and differentiation. This hypothesis was strengthened further when some of these genes were shown to encode growth factors or growth factor receptors. For example, the c-*sis* proto-oncogene encodes the B chain of platelet derived growth factor (PDGF) (Waterfield et al., 1983), while the c-*erbB* and c-*fms* proto-oncogenes encode the receptors for epidermal growth factor (EGF) (Downward et al., 1984) and monocyte-macrophage colony stimulating factor (M-CSF, or CSF-1)(Sherr et al., 1985), respectively. The Drosophila gene that encodes the EGF receptor homolog has been found recently to be allelic to *faint little ball*, a locus essential for embryonic development (Price et al., 1989; Schjter et al., 1989). The products of other oncogenes seem also to be part of the biochemical pathways by which a cell enters into S phase and mitosis after growth factor stimulation. *ras*, for example, encodes a cytoplasmic protein which is bound to the membrane and whose function might be related to the transduction of the mitotic signals induced by activation of growth factor receptors following the binding of their ligand. *raf* has also been implicated in the transmission of these signals to the nucleus: some growth factor receptors, such the PDGF receptor, activate c-*raf* protein through its direct binding and phosphorylation. The activation of the c-*raf* protein is followed by its translocation from the cytoplasm to the nucleus. Activated c-*raf*, which possess serine/threonine kinase activity, stimulates the activity of PEA1, a member of the c-*jun* oncogene family (Morrison et al., 1988; Rapp et al., 1989). Like the c-*fos* and c-*myc* products, the expression of the protein encoded by c-*jun*, located in the nucleus, is stimulated by different growth factors, including EGF (Quantin & Breathnach, 1988). The c-*jun* product forms a complex with the product of c-*fos*. Through its binding to critical sequences located in the promoter of different target genes, this complex functions as a transcriptional factor (AP1) regulating the expression of genes which are probably essential for the regulation of cell division (Rausscher et al., 1988). These data demonstrate the linkage between growth factor stimulation at cell periphery and transcriptional activation in the nucleus, leading to DNA synthesis and to cell transformation. Our review and our work concentrate on the events occurring at the cell membrane, and more especially, on the mechanisms and biological consequences of the EGF receptor activation.

THE EPIDERMAL GROWTH FACTOR RECEPTOR

The EGF receptor is a transmembrane glycoprotein that has a ligand dependent tyrosine kinase activity (Martin, 1986; Carpenter, 1987; Schlessinger, 1988a). Different growth factors are able to bind and activate the receptor. Among these ligands, two are predominant: the epidermal growth factor (EGF, also initially called β-urogastrone, 53 amino acids) and the transforming growth factor-alpha (TGFα, 50 amino acids), are generated by extracellular proteolytic cleavage of transmembrane precursors. They differ significantly in where they are produced. EGF, which is synthesized in the kidney and the salivary glands and found in almost all body fluids

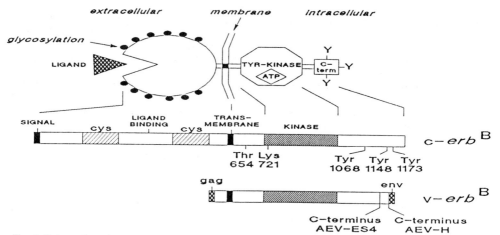

Fig. 1: Schematic representation of the full length and truncated EGF receptors encoded by the c-erbB and v-erbB oncogenes, respectively.

under normal physiological conditions, seems to function principally via an endocrine mode. TGFα is produced by normal (especially keratinocytes) and malignant cells, and appears to act locally via a paracrine, autocrine or juxtacrine mode (Wong et al., 1989). The EGF receptor is the only known receptor for these factors. Other ligands for the EGF receptor have been described: amphiregulin, isolated recently from serum-free conditioned medium of the MCF-7 human breast carcinoma cell line (Shoyab et al., 1989); and the poxvirus growth factors, especially vaccinia growth factor, whose presence is important to the virulence of the virus (Buller, 1988).

The mature EGF receptor is synthesized from a precursor (134 kDa) having a signal peptide at his N-terminus. After its cleavage, the resulting protein (131 kDa) is N-glycosylated (170 kDa). Its 1186 amino acid sequence contains three major regions (Fig. 1):
1) the N-terminal extracellular region (621 amino acids) is glycosylated and contains the binding domain (from the amino acids 294 to 543) of the receptor to the ligands, which is located between two cysteine rich sequences (Lax et al., 1988).
2) a single hydrophobic transmembrane region (23 amino acids).
3) the C-terminal intracellllular region (542 amino acids) contains the tyrosine kinase domain (243 amino acids, from the amino acids 694 to 937). Lysine residue 721 is essential for binding the ATP molecule that generates the phosphate for the phosphorylation reaction. This region also contains threonine 654, which is phosphorylated in vivo and in vitro by protein kinase C (phosphorylation of the receptor by this kinase is associated with a loss of the high affinity receptors and with a decrease in tyrosine kinase activity). At the C-terminus are located the three major sites of autophosphorylation: tyrosine residues (Tyr) 1068, 1148, and 1173.

In the absence of ligand, the receptors are distributed homogeneously on the cell membrane. After binding ligand, the receptors migrate to coated pits and are then internalized in endosomes. After fusion of these endosomes with lysosomes, the receptors and the ligands are rapidly degraded (Carpenter & Cohen, 1976). Numerous data are now available suggesting that the tyrosine kinase of the EGF receptor represents its effector function: this kinase activity has been shown to be essential for signal transduction, normal receptor trafficking, stimulation of DNA synthesis, and transformation (Honegger et al., 1987; Chen et al., 1987; Moolenaar et al., 1988). Studies of crosslinking experiments suggest that EGF activates the kinase activity of the EGF receptor by inducing its dimerization (Schlessinger, 1988b). Activation of the receptor kinase can nevertheless occur in the absence of receptor oligomerization (Northwood & Davis, 1988). Mutations of the transmembrane region do not affect EGF induced tyrosine kinase activity (Kashles et al., 1988). This observation is compatible with this model of receptor aggregation to explain how EGF binding stimulates its kinase activity, and not with a model invoking a conformational change transmitted through the membrane via the transmembrane fragment. Stimulation of the EGF receptor tyrosine kinase leads to its autophosphorylation and to phosphorylation of tyrosine residues from various cellular substrates, including p36 (one of the lipocortins), p42 (a protein phosphorylated in mitogen-stimulated cells), and the protein encoded by the neu oncogene (Gilmore et al., 1985; Brugge, 1986;

Stern & Kamps, 1988). Early responses to EGF receptor activation include a rise in cytoplasmic free Ca^{2+} and activation of the phosphoinositide-second messenger system in a variety of cell types (Carpenter, 1987). One of the substrates phosphorylated by the EGF receptor has been shown recently to be the Mr=145,000 form of the phospholipase C (PLC-II), enzyme inducing the phosphoinositide hydrolysis (Wahl et al, 1989). There is however no evidence that the presently identified substrates of the EGF receptor are the physiological mediators of the EGF induced mitogenic signal. Moreover, recent data suggest that these early responses are not sufficient, and maybe not even necessary, to elicit a mitogenic response to growth factors, which suggest that they could not be part of the biochemical cascade transmitting the mitogenic signal from the membrane to the nucleus (L'Allemain & Pouyssegur, 1986; Escobedo & Williams, 1988).

TRANSFORMING POTENTIAL OF THE EPIDERMAL GROWTH FACTOR RECEPTOR

1. N- and C-terminal truncations of the EGF receptor: the avian erythroblastosis viruses

The avian erythroblastosis viruses (AEV) contain the oncogene v-erbB, which is the gene principally responsible for their tumorigenic activity (erythroleukemias and fibrosarcomas). v-erbB, like all the retroviral oncogenes, was derived by transduction of a normal cellular gene, the c-erbB proto-oncogene, which encodes the EGF receptor. v-erbB differs from c-erbB by deletions of both the 5' and the 3' ends, resulting in the lost of the extracellular region and of one (strain AEV-H) or two (strain AEV-ES4, containing a second oncogene: v-erbA) major autophosphorylation sites of the EGF receptor. v-erbB also differs from c-erbB by point mutations which introduce some amino acid substitutions into the v-erbB product. Because of the N-terminal truncation, the v-erbB product does not contain any ligand binding domain, and, consequently, is not downregulated (internalized), in contrast to activated normal EGF receptors. Its transforming activity seems to result from a constitutive activation of its tyrosine kinase activity (Martin, 1986).

2. Full-length EGF receptor: potential role in human cancers

Several different human cancers frequently contain high levels of apparently normal EGF receptors. These tumors include principally glioblastoma and epidermoid epitheliomas of the lung, cervix, breast, head, and neck. Similar overexpression has been found in various cell lines derived from these tumors, for example the A418, SCC-15 and MDA-468 cell lines. Some tumor cells display more than 2 millions EGF receptors per cell. This overexpression is frequently the consequence of gene amplification, with sometimes more than 100 copies per cell. Their epidermoid origin seems to be quite characteristic. While epidermoid epithelioma of the lung, for example, is characterized by such an overexpression, lung tumors of other origin contain typically other activated oncogenes: K-ras (point mutation) in the adenocarcinoma and c-myc (amplification) in the small-cell carcinoma. The presence and the degree of c-erbB overexpression has been associated, in several studies, with a higher malignancy of these tumors, as estimated by their degree of invasiveness and of differentiation, the frequency of their relapse, and the survival of the patients (Neal et al., 1985; Sainsbury et al., 1987). Since the constitutive activation of the tyrosine kinase activity of the v-erbB product seems to be responsible for the tumorigenic potential of the avian erythroblastosis viruses, it was tempting to hypothesize that an increased tyrosine kinase activity resulting from the overexpression of the normal EGF receptor observed in human cancers, might also contribute to tumorigenesis. To test this hypothesis, we inserted a normal human EGF receptor cDNA (EGFR) from A431 cells into a retroviral vector (Velu et al., 1987). NIH 3T3 cells transfected with the viral DNA or infected with the corresponding rescued hEGFR retrovirus expressed high levels of normal human EGF receptors (400,000 human EGF receptors per cell) and developed a fully transformed phenotype in vitro that required both functional EGFR expression and the presence of EGF in the growth medium. Using different retroviral vectors, the transforming potential of the EGF receptor was found to depend upon the level of its expression, as well as on ligand concentration (Velu et al., 1989a). Cells expressing high level EGF receptors formed tumors in male nude mice, which produce significant amount of endogenous EGF, while control cells did not. Tumor development was much faster when exogenous EGF was administered to the mice. It was concluded that high levels of human EGF receptors can induce ligand dependent transformation and contribute to tumorigenicity (Velu et al., 1987). The ability of an overexpressed normal EGF receptor to induce EGF dependent NIH 3T3 cell transformation has been independently confirmed by others (Di Fiore et al., 1987; Riedel et al., 1988). To study the contribution of autocrine stimulation in cellular transformation, we used the hEGFR virus that we generated and which had a titer on NIH 3T3 cells that was higher than 10^7 focus-forming units per milliliter. hEGFR virus infection of NIH 3T3 cells previously transfected with a TGFα expression plasmid induced EGF-independent cell transformation. These results correlate with the frequent production of TGFα by several human tumor cells, like breast cancer cells, which also overexpressed EGF receptors (Derynck et al., 1987).

Most cancers with EGF receptor overexpression are of epidermoid origin, and we have found that the transforming potential of the hEGFR retrovirus was not limited to cells from fibroblastic origin (NIH 3T3 cells): viral infection of the mouse epithelial cell line C127, also conferred cell focal transformation and growth in agar. These studies provide direct experimental support for the hypothesis that increased numbers of EGF receptors can contribute to oncogenicity. The accessibility of the EGF receptor on the cell membrane and its dependence on a ligand for activity make it a potentially attractive target for therapy. Different molecules able to inhibit the EGF receptor are under study. Monoclonal antibodies directed against EGF receptor have shown anti-tumor activity against several carcinoma cells, in vitro and in nude mice (Masui et al., 1986). Tyrosine protein kinase inhibitors blocking EGF-dependent cell proliferation are also being developed (Yaish et al., 1988).

3. N- or C-terminal truncations of the EGF receptor

The normal EGF receptor, encoded by the c-erbB proto-oncogene, is subject to more stringent regulation than the product of the v-erbB oncogene, which is constitutively active. Several lines of evidence suggested that the C-terminus of the normal protein might serve an important negative regulatory function: 1) v-src, v-fms, and v-erbB, which are three viral oncogenes coding for tyrosine kinases, do not encode the last few C-terminal amino acids of the normal protein, and the deleted sequences invariably included the C-terminal tyrosine residue of the normal protein; 2) Previous reports have demonstrated that the C termini of the c-src and c-fms products negatively regulate their biological activity and that this effect is mediated by their C-terminal tyrosine residue. To determine whether this was true for the human EGF receptor, we have introduced two premature termination mutations in its coding sequences. These mutations result in deletion of one or two C-terminal tyrosine residues. Analogous truncations of the avian egfr gene are found in the v-erbB gene of the avian erythroblastosis viruses. The two C-terminal mutants induced EGF dependent cell transformation, but they were quantitatively less efficient than the gene encoding the full-length receptor (Velu et al., 1989b). In contrast to the results obtained with c-src and c-fms, these observations show that the extreme C-terminus of hEGFR does not have a negative function. Rather, it may facilitate transmission of the EGF receptor dependent signals for cell proliferation. These results imply that not all C-termini of tyrosine kinases function similarly, despite apparent structural similarities. The C-terminus of the EGF receptor contains three conserved Tyr (Y-1068, Y-1148, and Y-1173), which are autophosphorylated when the receptor is activated by EGF. To clarify their role, each Tyr was mutated separately to Phe, and studied as single, double, and triple mutants in the full length receptor. Analysis of these mutants indicated that the positive regulatory function of the C-terminus was principally mediated by the two C-terminal tyrosines, probably via autophosphorylation. The finding that premature termination of the human EGF receptor reduces its biological activity may appear paradoxal in view of its deletion in the receptors encoded by v-erbB. In these altered receptors, N-terminal truncation is the critical feature of the v-erbB encoded protein, leading by itself to the constitutive (EGF independent) activation of the receptor and is sufficient to render the gene capable of inducing erythroblastosis (Gamett et al., 1986; Khazaie et al., 1988; Wells & Bishop, 1988). C-terminal truncation has been shown principally to expand the tumorigenic host range to include sarcomas. Although many human tumors overexpress the full-length EGF receptor and the receptor in many avian tumors lacks its C-terminus, no tumors in any species have been identified in which C-terminal truncation of the cellular gene has occurred without N-terminal truncation. These considerations and other recent data (Haley et al., 1989) suggest that the biological consequences of C-terminal truncation of the EGF receptor may depend upon the integrity of the receptor N-terminus, with C-terminal deletion decreasing biological activity when the N-terminus is intact and increasing the activity when it is deleted.

ACTIVATION OF THE EGF RECEPTOR BY THE BOVINE PAPILLOMAVIRUS E5 TRANSFORMING PROTEIN

Recent studies that we performed suggest that another potential relation between EGF receptor and tumorigenesis could be its activation by the papillomavirus E5 transforming protein. Papillomavirus are the etiological agents of benign epithelial tumors (warts) and have been highly associated with certain epithelial malignancies of animals and humans, including cancer of the uterine cervix (Broker & Botchan, 1986). E5 is a major transforming gene for bovine papillomavirus (BPV), which induces fibropapillomas in its natural host. The 44 amino acid BPV E5 protein product localizes to cytoplasmic membrane, including the plasma membrane. In our studies of the mechanism by which this small peripheral protein might induce cellular transformation, we have found that BPV E5 can stimulate the activity of EGF receptors and CSF-1 receptors. When introduces into NIH 3T3 cells, normal human EGF receptors (encoded by c-erbB) and CSF-1 receptors (encoded by c-fms) can confer ligand dependent cell transformation, but there is no detectable activity without ligand. However, these receptors can cooperate with E5 to induce cell transformation in both the absence and the presence of ligand.

The cooperation between E5 and the growth factors receptors has some specificity in that two other cellular tyrosine kinases which are not growth factor receptors, c-*src* and c-*fes*, do not cooperate with E5. Analysis of EGF receptors in cells that contain E5 indicates that E5 induces a significant prolongation of receptor half-life in the presence or absence of ligand. This longer receptor half-life, which appears to be mediated via an E5 dependent inhibition of the normal pathway by which receptors are internalized and inactivated, seems to contribute significantly to the greater activity of the receptors in the presence of E5.

We conclude that, in addition to the constitutive activation of the truncated EGF receptors encoded by v-*erbB*, and to the EGF dependent activation of an overexpressed full length EGF receptors, bovine papillomavirus E5 protein can activate the normal human EGF receptor, probably by inhibiting receptor down-modulation.

REFERENCES

Bishop J.M. (1987): The molecular genetics of cancer. *Science* 235, 305-311.

Broker T.R. & Botchan, M. (1986): Papillomavirus: retrospectives and prospectives. In Cancer Cells: *DNA Tumor Viruses*, pp. 17-36. Cold Spring Harbor Laboratory, Cold Spring Harbor, New York.

Brugge J.S. (1986): The p35/p36 substrates of protein-tyrosine kinases as inhibitors of phospholipase A2. *Cell* 46, 149-150.

Buller R.M., Chakrabarti S., Cooper J.A., Twardzik D.R. & Moss B. (1988): Deletion of the vaccinia virus growth factor gene reduces virus virulence. *J. Virol.* 62, 866-874.

Carpenter G. & Cohen S. (1976): ^{125}I-labeled human epidermal growth factor: binding, internalization, and degradation in human fibroblasts. *J. Cell. Biol.* 71, 159-171.

Carpenter G. (1987): Receptors for egf and other polypeptide mitogens. *Annu. Rev. Biochem.* 56, 881-914.

Chen W.S., Lazar C.S., Poenie M., Tsien R.Y., Gill R.Y. & Rosenfeld G.M. (1987): Requirement for intrinsic protein tyrosine kinase activity in the immediate and late actions of the epidermal growth factor receptor. *Nature* 328, 820-823.

Derynck R., Goeddel D.V., Ullrich A., Gutterman J.U., Williams R.D., Bringman T.S. & Berger W.H. (1987): Synthesis of messenger RNAs for transforming growth factors alpha and beta and the epidermal growth factor receptor by human tumors. *Cancer Res.*: 47, 707-712.

Di Fiore P.P., Pierce J.H., Fleming T.P., Hazan R., Ullrich A., King C.R., Schlessinger J. & Aaronson S.A. (1987): Overexpression of the human epidermal growth factor receptor confers an EGF-dependent transformed phenotype to NIH 3T3 cells. *Cell* 51, 1063-1070.

Downward J., Yarden Y., Mayes E., Scrace G., Totty N., Stockwell P., Ullrich A., Schlessinger J. & Waterfield M. (1984): Close similarity of epidermal growth factor receptor and v-*erbB* oncogene protein sequences. *Nature* 307, 521-527.

Escobedo J.A. & Williams L.T. (1988): A PDGF receptor domain essential for mitogenesis but not for many other responses to PDGF. *Nature* 335, 85-87.

Gamett D.C., Tracy S.E. & Robinson H.L. (1986): Differences in sequences encoding the carboxy-terminal domain of the epidermal growth factor receptor correlate with differences in the disease potential of viral *erbB* genes. *Proc. Natl. Acad. Sci. USA* 83, 6053-6057.

Gilmore T., DeClue J.E. & Martin G.S. (1985): Protein phosphorylation at tyrosine is induced by the v-*erbB* gene product in vivo and in vitro. *Cell* 40, 609-618.

Haley J.D., Hsuan J.J. & Waterfield M.D. (1989): Analysis of mammalian fibroblast transformation by normal and mutated human epidermal growth factor receptors. *Oncogene* 4, 273-283.

Honegger A.M., Dull T.J., Felder S., Van Obberghen E., Bellot F., Szapary D., Schmidt A., Ullrich A. & Schlessinger J. (1987): Point mutation at the ATP binding site of epidermal growth factor receptor abolishes protein-tyrosine kinase activity and alters cellular routing. *Cell* 51, 199-209.

Kashles O., Szapary D., Bellot F., Ullrich A., Schlessinger J. & Schmidt A. (1988): Ligand-induced stimulation of epidermal growth factor receptor mutants with altered transmembrane regions. *Proc. Natl. Acad. Sci. USA* 85, 9567-9571.

Khazaie K., Dull T.J., Graf T., Schlessinger J., Ullrich A., Beug H. & Vennstrm B. (1988): Truncation of the human epidermal growth factor receptor leads to differential transforming potentials in primary avian fibroblasts and erythroblasts. *EMBO J.* 7, 3061-3071.

L'Allemain G. & Pouyssegur J. (1986): Epidermal growth factor and insulin action in fibroblasts: Evidence that phosphoinositide hydrolysis is not an essential mitogenic signalling pathway. *FEBS Lett.* 197, 344-348.

Lax I., Burgess W.H., Bellot F., Ullrich A., Schlessinger J. & Givol D. (1988): Localization of a major receptor-binding domain for epidermal growth factor by affinity labeling. *Mol. Cell. Biol.* 8, 1831-1834.

Martin G.S. (1986): The *erbB* gene and the epidermal growth factor receptor. *Cancer Surveys* 5, 199-219.

Masui H., Moroyama T. & Mendelsohn J. (1986): Mechanism of antitumor activity in mice for anti-epidermal growth factor receptor monoclonal antibodies with different isotypes. *Cancer Res.* 46, 5592-5598.

Moolenaar W.H., Bierman A.J., Tilly B.C., Verlaan I., Honegger A.M., Ullrich A. & Schlessinger J. (1988): A point mutation at the ATP-binding site of the epidermal growth factor receptor abolishes signal transduction. *EMBO J.* 7, 707-710.

Morrison D.K., Kaplan D.R., Rapp U. & Roberts T.M. (1988): Signal transduction from membrane to cytoplasm: growth factors and membrane-bound oncogene products increase *raf*-1 phosphorylation and associated protein kinase activity. *Proc. Natl. Acad. Sci. USA* 85: 8855-8859.

Neal D.E., Marsh C., Bennett M.K., Abel P.D., Hall R.R., Sainsbury J.R. & Harris A.L. (1985): Epidermal growth factor receptor in human bladder cancer: comparison of invasive and superficial tumors. *Lancet* 1, 366-368.

Northwood I.C. & Davis R.J. (1988): Activation of the epidermal growth factor receptor tyrosine kinase in the absence of receptor oligomerization. *J. Biol. Chem.* 263, 7450-7453.

Price J.V. & Clifford R.J. (1989): The maternal ventralizing locus *torpedo* is allelic to *faint little ball*, an embryonic lethal, and encodes the Drosophila EGF receptor homolog. *Cell* 56, 1085-1092.

Quantin B. & Breathnach R. (1988): Epidermal growth factor stimulates transcription of the c-*jun* proto-oncogene in rat fibroblasts. *Nature* 334, 538-539.

Rapp U.R., Heidecker G., Storm S., Wasylyk B., Anderson W., Siegel J., Klausner R., Morrison D., Williams L.T. & Roberts T. (1989): Role of *raf*-family protein kinases in mitogen signal transduction. In: *Abstract book, The Molecular Basis of Cell Growth Regulation.* NATO/EEC Course, Mallorca, Spain.

Rauscher III F.J., Cohen D.R., Curran T., Bos T.J., Vogt P.K., Bohmann P., Tjian R. & Franza B.R. (1988): *fos*-associated protein p39 is the product of the *jun* proto-oncogene. *Science* 240, 1010-1016.

Riedel H., Massoglia S., Schlessinger J. & Ullrich A. (1988): Ligand activation of overexpressed epidermal growth factor receptors transforms NIH 3T3 mouse fibroblasts. *Proc. Natl. Acad. Sci. USA* 85, 1477-1481.

Sainsbury J.R.C., Farndon J.R., Needham G.K., Malcolm A.J. & Harris A.L. (1987): Epidermal growth factor receptor status as predictor of early recurrence of and death from breast cancer. *Lancet* 1, 1398-1402.

Schejter E.D. & Shilo B.-Z. (1989): The Drosophila EGF receptor homolog (DER) gene is allelic to *faint little ball*, a locus essential for embryonic development. *Cell* 56, 1093-1104.

Schlessinger J. (1988a): The epidermal growth factor receptor as a multifunctional allosteric protein. *Biochemistry* 27, 3119-3123.

Schlessinger J. (1988b): Signal transduction by allosteric receptor oligomerization. *TIBC* 13, 443-447.

Sherr C.J., Rettenmier C.W., Sacca R., Roussel M.F., Look A.T. & Stanley E.R. (1985): The c-*fms* proto-oncogene product is related to the receptor for the mononuclear phagocyte growth factor, CSF-1. *Cell* 41, 665-676.

Shoyab M., Plowman G.D., McDonald V.L., Bradley J.G. & Todaro G.J. (1989): Structure and function of human amphiregulin: a member of the epidermal growth factor family. *Science* 243, 1074-1076.

Stern D.F. & Kamps M.P. (1988): Epidermal growth factor-stimulated tyrosine phosphorylation of p185^{neu}: a potential model for receptor interactions. *EMBO J.* 7, 995-1001.

Velu T.J., Beguinot L, Vass W.C., Willingham M.C., Merlino G.T., Pastan I. & Lowy D.R. (1987): Epidermal growth factor dependent transformation by a human EGF receptor proto-oncogene. *Science* 238, 1408-1410.

Velu T.J., Beguinot L, Vass W.C., Zhang K., Pastan I. & Lowy D.R. (1989a): Retroviruses expressing different levels of the normal epidermal growth factor receptor: biological properties and new bioassay. *J. Cell. Bioch.* 39, 153-166.

Velu T.J., Vass W.C., Lowy D.R. & Beguinot L. (1989b): Functional heterogeneity of proto-oncogene tyrosine kinases: the C terminus of the human epidermal growth factor receptor facilitates cell proliferation. *Mol. Cell. Biol.* 9, 1772-1778.

Wahl M.I., Nishibe S., Suh P., Rhee S.G. & Carpenter G. (1989): Epidermal growth factor stimulates tyrosine phosphorylation of phospholipase C-II independently of receptor internalization and extracellular calcium. *Proc. Natl. Acad. Sci. USA* 86, 1568-1572.

Waterfield M.D., Scrace G.T., Wittle N., Stroobant P., Johnsson A., Wasteson A., Westermark B., Heldin C.-H., Huang J.S. & Deuel T.F. (1983): Platelet-derived growth factor is structurally related to the putative transforming protein p28sis of simian sarcoma virus. *Nature* 304, 35-39.

Wells A. & Bishop J.M. (1988): Genetic determinants of neoplastic transformation by the retroviral oncogene v-*erbB. Proc. Natl. Acad. Sci. USA* 85, 7597-7601.

Wong S.T., Winchell L.F., McCune B.K., Earp H.S., Teixidc J., Massagu J., Herman B. & Lee D.C. (1989): The TGFα precursor expressed on the cell surface binds to the epidermal growth factor receptor on adjacent cells, leading to signal transduction. *Cell* 56, 495-506.

Yaish P., Gazit A., Gilon C. & Levitzki A. (1988): Blocking of epidermal growth factor-dependent cell proliferation by EGF receptor kinase inhibitors. *Science* 242, 933-935.

Hormones and Cell Regulation. N° 14, Eds J. Nunez, J.E. Dumont. Colloque INSERM/J. Libbey Eurotext Ltd. © 1989. Vol. 198, pp. 71-75

Microglial cell functions during brain development

Michel Mallat, Brigitte Chamak, Clotilde Thery and Danièle Leroy*

*INSERM U114, Chaire de neuropharmacologie, Collège de France, 11 Place Marcelin Berthelot, 75231 Paris Cedex 05, France and *Centre de recherche de Vitry-sur-Seine, Rhône-Poulenc Santé, 13 quai Jules Guesdes, 94407 Vitry sur Seine, France*

SUMMARY

Microglial cells constitute a population of the central nervous system (CNS) which displays some of the phenotypic features of tissue macrophages. These cells are involved in the regressive events of neurogenesis : They contribute to the elimination of degenerating cell bodies or neuronal processes.

Microglial cells, purified from rodent glial cultures, have been shown to release growth factors, such as interleukin 1 (IL 1) and nerve growth factor (NGF), wich act on astrocytes or neurons. These results suggest that in addition to phagocytic functions, microglial cells may exert a trophic role during ontogenesis.

INTRODUCTION

The term of microglia was first introduced in the early part of the century by del Rio Hortega (1932) when he specifically identified this cell population of the central nervous system (CNS) by a weak silver carbonate stain. Recent investigations have illustrated the participation of microglial cells in various processes. Within a neuroimmunological context microglia may behave like immunoeffector cells involved in local inflammatory responses (Giulian, 1987). Microglial cells also have appear as target cells for the human immunodeficiency virus in cases of AIDS associated encephalopathy (Budka, 1989). Functions of these cells related to CNS ontogenesis will here be reviewed following a brief outline on microglial phenotypes.

MICROGLIAL PHENOTYPES

In the adult rat CNS microglial cells account for 5 to 10 % of the neuroglial cells . They display a small cell body with long branched and crenellated processes (Ling, 1981). Several markers, common to tissue macrophages, were recently found to be expressed by microglial cells of rodents (Perry et al, 1985). These observations further support the most widely accepted view about the microglial lineage whereby these cells would stem from the invasion of the immature CNS by blood monocytes (Ling, 1980). In the developing CNS, microglial cells display a phenotype more akin to macrophages involved in an inflammatory response. This phenotype was quoted under many terms such as ameboid microglia or brain macrophages. Contrasting with the "ramified" cells of the adult tissue, ameboid microglial cells have a copious cytoplasm in which phagosomes and abundant lysosomes can be seen. Several macrophages markers were used to map these cells in the developing CNS. Ameboid microglial cells were readily detected in foetal brain of rats or mices at the 16th day of gestation. During postnatal stages, these cells are preferentially located in subcortical white matter; their progressive disappearance (completed in 3 week old rats) may result from cell death, migration out of the tissue or transformation into ramified microglial cells (for reviews and references see Ling, 1981; Perry & Gordon, 1988).

FUNCTIONS OF MICROGLIAL CELLS DURING CNS DEVELOPMENT

Ameboid microglia appear involved both in trophic and regressive events taking place during neurogenesis.

I. Microglia and regressive events of neurogenesis

Massive waves of neuronal death were observed in multiple structures of the developing CNS. This ontogenetic phenomenon is considered as a way of regulating the specificity and the number of connections made between nerve cells and their targets (Cowan et al., 1984). Histological observations have enlighted the phagocytic behavior of ameboid microglia ; its contribution to the withdrawal of degenerating neurons was shown in different regions of the CNS (Hume et al., 1983; Perry et al., 1985). The accumulation of ameboid microglia cells in specific subcortical structures was also correlated with macrophagic tasks. Hankin et al. (1988) have shown that the phagocytosis of dying astroglial cells, located beneath the Corpus Callosum, participates to the formation of an intracerebral cavity : the Cavum Septum Pellucidum. Later during the development, the presence of ameboid microglial cells is also coincident with the removal of misdirected or exuberant axons from living neurons. Ultrastructural evidences have supported the notion that these ameboid microglial cells might be involved in the elimination of transitory axons which do not display obvious signs of degeneration (Innocenti et al., 1983 ab). Thus the question was raised whether specific signals could trigger the recognition of appropriate targets for local phagocytosis (Killackey, 1984). The existence of such signals remains to be demonstrated. However it is known that the phagocytic behavior of tissue macrophages can be directed and stimulated by different molecules including antibodies or compounds generated by complement activation (C3 sub-fragments) (Wright & Silverstein, 1986). Receptors for these compounds are expressed by microglial cells (Perry & Gordon., 1985). Thus we have investigated the availability of complement compounds in the developing brain using in vitro primary cultures of embryonic glial or neuronal cells and immortalized astrocytic cell lines. Immunoprecipitations of newly synthetized proteins and Northern blot detection of mRNA have demonstrated the astrocytic production of factor B and C3, the two key compounds involved in the alternative pathway of complement activation (Levi-Strauss & Mallat, 1987). Although the in vivo occurence of complement activation in the developing brain remains to be explored, the above results suggest a functional cooperation between microglial cells and astrocytes during regressive events. Synergistic interactions with astrocytes extend to other aspects of microglial functions such as trophic influences.

II. Trophic functions of ameboid microglia

Studies of microglial functions have substantially benefited from recent methods for in vitro purification and culture of rodent microglial cells (Frei et al., 1986; Giulian & Baker, 1985). These cells were recovered from primary glial cultures obtained from embryos or neonates. They were purified by selective adhesion to refractory substrates such as plastic or glass. The adherent cells fulfilled the criteria for in situ identification of ameboid microglia (Fig 1 ; Mallat et al., 1989). Their proliferation was shown to be stimulated by purified colony-stimulating factors (CSFs) acting on myeloid lineages such as interleukin 3 (IL3), granulocyte/macrophage CSF (GM-CSF) and macrophage-CSF (M-CSF) (Giulian et al., 1988).

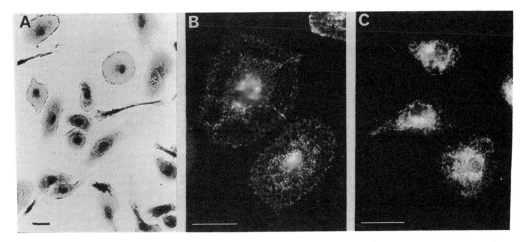

Fig. 1: Purified ameboid microglial cells derived from rat embryonic mesencephalon, two days after isolation. A: toluidin blue staining. B & C: immunofluorescent staining; B: monoclonal antibody (Mab) OX42 against the receptor to the iC3b fragment of the complement C3 molecule; C: Mab ED1 against an intracytoplasmic antigen specific of macrophages (Sminia et al., 1987). Scale bar: 25 µm

II.a. Mitogenic interactions between astrocytes and microglial cells

New insights into microglial functions stemmed from the detection of soluble growth factors in these cultures. The microglial release of mitogenic peptides acting on astrocytes was first evidenced by Giulian and Baker (1985). Among these peptides, the immunomodulator Interleukin 1 (IL 1) was detected using specific bioassays (mitogenic effects on mouse thymocytes or D-10 cell line). The in vitro release of IL 1 by microglial cells was induced by macrophage activators such as lipopolysaccharides (LPS) (Giulian et al., 1986). We have extended this observation by showing that LPS stimulate the transcription of both α and β IL 1 genes in mouse microglial cell cultures (Hetier et al., 1988).

Purified IL 1 was shown to stimulate mitosis of astrocytes both *in vivo* and *in vitro* (Giulian & Lachman, 1985). In addition, IL 1 biological activity was monitored by the thymocyte assay in extracts collected from cerebral cortex or cerebellum at different periods during ontogenesis. Amount of IL 1 appeared to correlate with the number of ameboid cells detected in the freshly dissociated tissues. Altogether, these results led Giulian et al. (1988) to propose that ameboid microglia regulates astroglial growth within specific sites of the developing brain.

Conversely, astrocytes might favor the development of the microglial cell population. In fact, *in vitro* outgrowth of ameboid microglia was clearly observed on confluent glial layers enriched in astrocytes. Moreover, astrocytes, stimulated with LPS, have been shown to release soluble factors which increase microglial mitoses and display IL3-like biological activities (Frei et al., 1985). An eventual production of IL 3 in the CNS was further confirmed by detection of IL 3 mRNA in the adult mouse brain (Farrar et al., 1989). In addition, we have recently evidenced the production of M-CSF by a murin astrocytic cell line (MES 3-1) by performing Northern Blot analyses. Thus various growth factors, including known CSFs, might account for a mitogenic influence of astrocytes on microglial cells.

II.b. microglial production of NGF

Through the enhancement of astroglial growth, microglia may indirectly influence the neuronal development which is widely regulated by astrocytes (Chamak et al., 1988). Nevertheless, we took advantage of the cultures to look for a microglial production of neurotrophic factors such as the NGF. This polypeptide was detected in cultures of rat microglial cells by using an immunoenzymatic assay. Its release into the culture medium was strongly induced by treating the cells with LPS. This microglial response to LPS possibly illustrate a functional specialization of CNS phagocytes since at best, only small amounts of NGF were recovered from cultivated peritoneal macrophages used for comparison (Mallat et al., 1989). Given the effects of NGF in the CNS (for review see Korshing, 1986), these results suggest that in addition to sub populations of neurons or astrocytes (Lindsay, 1979 ; Whittemore et al., 1988), ameboid microglia also might favor the maturation and the survival of central cholinergic neurons. NGF production by perivascular microglia might also contribute to the development of the sympathetic innervation of CNS blood vessels .

CONCLUSIONS

The actual data suggest an active and diversified participation of ameboid microglia to the CNS histogenesis. The involvment of microglia in cellular regressive events may not be limited to the elimination of dead cells, considering a possible phagocytosis of axonal processes from living neurons. *In vitro* purification of microglial cells will help to clarify these interactions with neuronal processes. Meanwhile, based on the detection of growth factor secretions, microglial cultures have led to postulate trophic functions for these cells. However, the microglial production of growth factors (IL1, NGF) was mainly observed upon stimulations of the cells with classical macrophagic activators (LPS) unrelated to the CNS development. Endogenous microglial activators remain to be found. For this purpose, Investigations can rely on the extensive data obtained with macrophages from various tissues. In particular, extracellular matrix compounds or neuropeptides should be considered in light of their reported effects on peripheral macrophages.(Beezhold & Lause, 1987; Hartung et al., 1986)

REFERENCES

Beezhold, D.H. & Lause, D.B. (1987): Stimulation of rat macrophage Interleukin 1 secretion by plasma fibronectin. Immunol. Invest. 16, 437-449.
Budka, H. (1989): Human immunodeficiency virus (HIV)-induced disease of the central nervous system: pathology and implications for pathogenesis. Acta Neuropathol. 77, 225- 236.
Chamak, B. Fellous, A., Glowinski, J. & Prochiantz, A. (1987): MAP2 expression and neuritic outgrowth and branching are coregulated through region-specific neuro-astroglial interactions. J. Neurosci. 7, 3163-3170.
Cowan, W.M., Fawcett, J.W., O'Leary, D.D.M. & Stanfield, B.B. (1984): Regressive events in neurogenesis. Science 225, 1258-1265.
del Rio Hortega, P. (1932): Microglia. In *Cytology and Cellular Pathology of the Nervous system*, ed W. Penfield, pp. 481-534. New York: Paul B. Hoeber.
Frei, K., Bodmer, S., Schwerdel, C. & Fontana, A. (1986): Astrocytes derived interleukine 3 as a growth factor for microglial cells and peritoneal macrophages. J. Immunol. 137, 3521-3527.
Giulian D. & Lachman, L.L.B. (1985): Interleukin-1 stimulation of astroglial proliferation after brain injury. Science 228, 497-499.
Giulian, D. & Baker, T.J. (1985): Peptides released by ameboid microglia stimulate astroglial proliferation. J. Cell. Biol. 101, 2411-2415.
Giulian, D., Young, D.G., Woodward, J., Brown, D.C., & Lachman, L.B. (1986): Interleukin-1 of the central nervous system is produced by ameboid microglia. J. Exp. Med. 164, 594-604.
Giulian, D. (1987): Ameboid microglia as effectors of inflammation in the central nervous system. J. Neurosci. Res. 18 , 155-171.
Giulian, D., Vaca, K. & Johnson, B. (1988a): Secreted peptides as regulators of neuron-glia and glia-glia interactions in the developing nervous system. J. Neurosci. Res. 21, 487-500.
Hankin, M.H., Schneider, B.F. & Silver, J. (1988): Death of the subcallosal glial sling is

correlated with formation of the Cavum Septi Pellucidi. J. Comp. Neurol. 272, 191-202.

Hartung, H.P., Wolters, K. & Toyka, K.U. (1986): Substance P: binding properties and studies on cellular responses in guinea pig macrophages. J. Immunol. 136, 3856-3863.

Hetier, E., Ayala, J., Denèfle, P., Bousseau, A., Rouget, P., Mallat, M. & Prochiantz, A. (1988): Brain macrophages synthesize interleukin 1 and interleukin 1 mRNA in vitro. J. Neurosci. Res. 21, 391-397.

Hume, D.A., Perry, V.H. & Gordon, S. (1983): Immunohistochemical localization of a macrophage specific antigen in the developing mouse retina: phagocytosis of dying neurons and differenciation of microglial cells to form a regular array in the plexiform layers. J. Cell. Biol. 97, 253-257.

Innocenti, G.M., Koppel, H. & Clarke, S. (1983a): Transitory macrophages in the white matter of the developing visual cortex. I -Light and electron microscopic characteristics and distribution. Dev. Brain Res. 11, 39-53.

Innocenti, G.M., Koppel, H. & Clarke, S. (1983b): Transitory macrophages in the visual cortex. II. Development and relations with axonal pathways. Dev. Brain Res. 11, 55-66.

Killackey, H.P. (1984): Glia and the elimination of transient cortical projections. TINS 7, 225- 226.

Korsching, S. (1986): The role of nerve growth factor in the CNS. TINS 9, 570-573.

Lévi-Strauss, M. & Mallat, M. (1987): Primary cultures of murine astrocytes produce C3 and factor B components of the alternative pathway of complement activation. J. Immunol. 139, 2361-2366.

Lindsay, R.M. (1979): Adult rat brain astrocytes support survival of both NGF-dependent and NGF-insensitive neurons. Nature 282, 80-82.

Ling, E.A., Don Penney & Leblond, C.P. (1980): Use of carbon labeling to demonstrate the role of blood monocytes as precursors of the "ameboid cells" in the corpus callosum of post-natal rats. J. Comp. Neur. 193, 631-657.

Ling, E.A. (1981): The origin and nature of microglia. In *Advances in cellular neurobiology*, ed. S. Fedoroff & L. Hertz, vol.2, 33-82. New York: Academic Press.

Mallat, M., Houlgatte, R., Brachet, P. & Prochiantz, A. (1989): Lipopolysaccharide-stimulated rat brain macrophages release NGF in vitro. Dev. Biol. 133, 309-311.

Perry, V.H., Hume, D.A. & Gordon, S. (1985): Immmunohistochemical localization of macrophages and microglia in the developing and adult mouse brain. Neuroscience 15,313-326.

Perry, V.H. & Gordon, S. (1988): Macrophages and microglia in the nervous system. TINS 11, 273-277.

Sminia, T., De Groot, C.J.A., Djikstra, C.D., Koetsier, J.C. & Polman, C.H. (1987): Macrophages in the central nervous system of the rat. Immmunobiol. 174, 43-50.

Whittemore, S.R., Friedman, P.L., Larhammar, D., Persson, HJ., Gonzalez-Carvajal, M. & Holets, V.R. (1988): Rat β-nerve growth factor sequence and site of synthesis in the adult hippocampus. J. Neurosci. Res. 20, 403-410.

Wright, S.D. & Silverstein, S.C. (1986): Overview: the function of receptors in phagocytosis. In *Handbook of experimental immunology*, ed. D.M. Weir, vol.2, chapter 41. Oxford: Alden Press.

RESUME

La microglie forme une sous population cellulaire du système nerveux central qui se distingue par l'expression de marqueurs des macrophages tissulaires. Ces cellules sont impliquées dans les évènements régressifs de la neurogenèse : elles participent à l'élimination de prolongements neuronaux ou de corps cellulaires en dégénérescence.

Les cellules microgliales de rongeurs ont été purifiées *in vitro* à partir de cultures gliales primaires issues d'animaux immatures. Elles se sont révélées sources de facteurs de croissance actifs sur des astrocytes ou des neurones (interleukine 1 ou NGF). Ces données sont en faveur d'un rôle trophique de la microglie qui s'ajouterait aux fonctions de phagocytose, au cours de l'ontogenèse.

75

Control mechanisms in other systems

Mécanismes de contrôle dans d'autres systèmes

Hormones and Cell Regulation. N° 14, Eds J. Nunez, J.E. Dumont. Colloque INSERM/J. Libbey Eurotext Ltd. © 1989. Vol. 198, pp. 79-83

Control of B cell activation in humans

A. Diu, M. Fevrier, P. Mollier and J. Thèze

Immunogénétique Cellulaire, Institut Pasteur, 28, rue du Dr Roux, Paris, France.

Abstract : We have been studying the interactions between T helper and B lymphocytes during T-B cell cooperation. In particular we have been trying to evaluate the respective role of direct cell to cell contact versus soluble factor mediated events during B lymphocyte activation. Some lymphokines were shown to play a role during the early phases of B cell activation. Interleukin-4 can induce changes in surface antigen-expression on resting B-cells but it does not induce by itself complete B cell activation. Interleukin-2 could also have some effects on resting B cells. In addition, we have described a system where resting B cells can be polyclonally activated by T cell derived soluble factors. We were able to show that cell to cell contact was not required and that soluble products distinct from IL-2 and IL-4 were sufficient to induce full B lymphocyte activation.

During the response to a T-dependent antigen, T helper cells which have been activated by processed antigen presented on "antigen-presenting cells" are thought to completely control the proliferation and clonal expansion of antigen-specific B cells as well as their differentiation into plasma cells. Helper T cells secrete many different lymphokines that are involved in the regulation of immune responses. In particular, several factors are implicated in the regulation of the humoral immune response leading to the production of specific antibodies against a given antigen. Lymphokines directed towards activated B lymphocytes have been characterized in the human system. They were shown to have different effects on B cell proliferation and/or differentiation and their study permits better understanding of the influence of T cells on B cell-responses.

However, for a humoral response to be elicited, a recognition step between antigen-specific T helper cells and B cells is needed. During this initial event, T helper cells recognize, by means of their specific receptor, the processed antigen expressed on the B cell surface in association with MHC class II molecules. This initial step results in activation of the antigen-specific B cell which becomes susceptible to T-cell derived factors inducing proliferation and differentiation. Little is known about the exact nature of the signal transmitted during T cell-B cell interaction. One can postulate two different mechanisms by which a helper T cell could act on a resting B cell : 1) cell-cell contact involving interaction between T cell receptor and MHC class II antigens on B cells and 2) lymphokine-mediated activation which does not require recognition of MHC class II determinants. At the early stage of B cell activation, the respective role of these two different mechanisms is still poorly understood.

In order to address this problem, we have been studying soluble factors which could be implicated in B cell activation. We will review here work from our laboratory and from others providing evidence that non-specific lymphokines can participate in the initial steps of B cell activation.

IL-4 is an activating-factor for human B cells

Human IL-4 was recently obtained in recombinant form by molecular cloning based on homology with a mouse IL-4 cDNA. It permits human B cell proliferation if appropriate pre-activation of the B cells is provided (anti-IgM coupled to Sepharose beads or Staphylococcus aureus Cowan A, SAC). Human IL-4 does not promote resting B cell proliferation but it was shown to act on resting B cells by inducing Fcε receptor expression. This effect involves 30 % of a B cell population and occurs in cells of high density and low RNA content corresponding to cells in G_0 phase.

Whether or not human IL-4 can increase HLA class II expression on human resting B cells remains controversial. Human IL-4 enhances HLA-DR and DQ expression in several Burkitt lymphoma cell lines but it was found not to affect HLA class II expression on normal human tonsilar or peripheral B cells. In addition, recent data from our laboratory suggest that human IL-4 has no effect on HLA class II antigen expression of normal human splenic B cells.

Although differences in target populations could explain the differences between murine and human IL-4, it remains true that, if Ia induction is the main feature of murine IL-4, Fcε receptor induction is a characteristic of human IL-4. None of the other B cell lymphokines alone or in conjunction with anti-Ig can induce Fcε receptor expression on B cells. The biological function of Fcε receptor is still unclear. A soluble form of the Fcε receptor is released from human B cells activated with IL-4 and this soluble Fcε receptor was shown to have B cell growth-promoting activities. In addition, IL-4 appears to be involved in the regulation of IgE synthesis by B cells since IgE secretion is observed when peripheral blood mononuclear cells are cultured with human IL-4. However, the IgE secretion-inducing effect of IL-4 is indirect and requires the presence of both T cells and monocytes. Since IL-4 can act on both T cells and monocytes, IgE synthesis by B cells is likely to result from a cascade of events involving other factors produced by these cells.

Is IL-2 an activation factor for B cells ?

IL-2 was initially described as a T-cell growth factor but it can also act as a growth factor and a differentiation factor for anti-Ig or SAC-preactivated human B lymphocytes. Activated human B cells express the high affinity IL-2 receptor and respond to IL-2 in conjunction with anti-Ig. However, when high concentrations of recombinant IL-2 are used, IL-2 can directly induce the proliferation of peripheral blood mononuclear cells as well as the differentiation of purified non-preactivated B cells. As postulated for resting T cells, this effect could be explained by the binding of IL-2 to the p70 subunit of the IL-2 receptor which can bind IL-2 with intermediate affinity. Although cne can postulate that very high local lymphokine concentrations can occur physiologically in the vicinity of activated T cells, some questions remain concerning the exact physiological role of IL-2 as an activating factor for resting human B cells.

Evidence for a human B-cell activating factor and its relationship to human IL-4 and IL-2

In extending our work on murine B cells, we have demonstrated that human T cell clones, after activation with anti-CD3 or anti-CD2 monoclonal antibodies release a soluble component of apparent m.w. 12-15 000 which induces the proliferation of highly purified resting human B cells. This activity was called human BCAF and its effects on B cells were shown to include :

induction of 4F2 antigen and transferrin receptor expression, cell volume enlargement, increase in HLA class II (DR, DP and DQ) antigen expression and finally, progression of the B cells through S phase and mitosis. As in the mouse system, these effects are not MHC-restricted and affect B cells that are in a resting state (G_0 phase of the cell cycle).

Our present efforts concentrate on characterizing and purifying the molecule(s) responsible for this activity. Although we are presently using crude T cell supernatants containing BCAF activity, it was possible to investigate its relationship to other lymphokines implicated in human B cell activation (and in particular IL-4 and IL-2) by using neutralising monoclonal antibodies directed against these lymphokines.

Human BCAF can induce the expression of p55 IL-2 receptors on 20 % of the B cells but IL-2 does not participate in the B cell proliferation induced by T cell supernatants containing both IL-2 and BCAF. This was demonstrated by neutralising IL-2 in supernatants with a specific monoclonal antibody or blocking the IL-2 receptor on B cells with anti-Tac monoclonal antibodies. In addition, we recently obtained T cell clones secreting BCAF activity in the absence of any detectable IL-2.

In a recent study, we establish that IL-4 does not participate in the different effects of BCAF-containing supernatants on resting B cells, including cell size enlargement, increase in HLA class II antigen expression and B cell proliferation. Inhibition of IL-4 activity in T cell supernatants by specific anti IL-4 antiserum does not diminish any of these effects on B cells. In addition, one T cell clone and a tumor T cell line can secrete BCAF without any detectable IL-4.

Using BCAF-containing supernatants free of IL-4, we were able to compare their effects on Fce receptor- expression to the effect of human IL-4. Human IL-4 can induce Fce receptor expression on 30 % of unstimulated splenic B cells whereas BCAF-containing supernatants do not induce Fce receptor expression while still promoting B cell proliferation. This observation further confirms that human BCAF and human IL-4 are distinct molecules. It also suggests that they activate resting human B cells via different pathways. IL-4 would preferentially drive resting B cells through an activation pathway involving Fce receptor expression and may be facilitating the immunoglobulin switch to IgE secretion. On the other hand, BCAF would induce a different activation pathway for resting B cells in which HLA class II antigen expression is enhanced but where B cells do not become sensitive to IL-2 or IL-4.

Conclusion

Interactions among cell-surface molecules play an important role during T cell - B cell cooperation. In particular, the T cell receptor is though to recognize processed antigen expressed in association with MHC class II molecules on B cells. Aside from these receptor-mediated interactions, growing evidence comes from the literature that lymphokines participate in the early steps of T cell controlled-B cell activation.

It now seems established that resting G_0 phase B cells can express functional receptors for lymphokines. Interleukin-4, first described in the murine system, is the best characterized activating factor directed towards B cells. However, it only induces partial activation of the resting B cells.

Work from this and other laboratories indicates that soluble factors distinct from IL-4 display activating properties on resting B cells. Although complete characterization of BCAF has not yet been achieved, partially purified preparations retain the capacity to induce full B cell activation and progression of the B cells from G_0 to S and M phases of the cell cycle. This suggests that one or several molecules can completely replace T helper cells in promoting resting B cell proliferation.

One can only speculate about the physiological significance of these non-specific activating molecules. They could be short-range acting factors that would only trigger those resting B cells that come in close contact with a T helper cell. Alternatively, these molecules could have a function in amplifying the immune rsponse by recruiting . more T and B cells and broadening the restricted antigen-specific antibody response.

References

Abbas A.K. (1988) : A reassessment of the mechanisms of antigen-specific T-cell dependent B-cell activation. Immunol. Today ; 9:89
Bich-Thuy L.T., Dukovich M. et al. (1987) : Direct activation of resting human T cells by IL-2: the role of an IL-2 receptor distinct from the Tac protein. J. Immunol. ; 139:1550
Bich-Thuy L.T., and Fauci A.S. (1985) : Direct effect of interleukin-2 on the differentiation of human B cells which have not been preactivated in vitro. Eur. J. Immunol. ; 15:1075
Diu A., Gougeon M.L. et al. (1987) : Activation of resting human B cells by T cell clone supernatant: characterization of a human B cell activating factor. Proc. Natl. Acad. Sci. USA ; 84:9140
Diu A. , Leclercq L. et al. (1987) : Supernatant from a cloned helper T cell stimulates resting B cells to express transferrin and IL-2 receptors. Cellular Immunology; 107:471
Leclercq L., Cambier J.C. et al. (1986) : Supernatant from a cloned helper T cell stimulates most small resting B cells to undergo increased I-A expression, blastogenesis, and progression through cell cycle. J. Immunol.; 136:539
O'Garra A., Umland S et al. (1988) : "B cell factors" are pleiotropic. Immunol. Today ; 9:47
Paul W.E., and Ohara J. (1987) : B-cell stimulatory factor-1/Interleukin-4. Ann. Rev. Immunol.; 5:429
Roth C., Moreau J.L. et al. (1988) : Biochemical characterization and biological effects of partially purified B cell activating factor (BCAF). Eur. J. Immunol. ; 18:577
Rousset F., de Waal Malefijt R. et al. (1988) : Regulation of Fc receptor for IgE (CD23) and class II MHC expression on Burkitt's lymphoma cell lines by human IL-4 and IFN-g. J. Immunol. ; 140:2625

Résumé Nous nous sommes intéressés à l'étude des rapports entre lymphocytes T auxiliaires et lymphocytes B au cours de la coopération T-B. Nous avons plus particulièrement tenté d'évaluer la part respective des interactions directes entre cellules par rapport aux facteurs solubles au cours de l'activation des lymphocytes B. Certains facteurs de type lymphokines peuvent agir au cours de l'activation précoce du lymphocyte B. L'interleukine 4, notamment, induit certains changements dans les antigènes de surface des lymphocytes B au repos mais elle ne permet pas à elle seule une activation complète du lymphocyte B. L'interleukine-2 pourrait également jouer un rôle à ce niveau. Enfin, nous avons mis au point un système d'activation polyclonale des lymphocytes B sous l'influence de facteurs issus des lymphocytes T. Nous avons pu montrer qu'un contact cellulaire n'était pas indispensable et que des produits solubles différents de l'IL-2 et de l'IL-4 suffisaient à induire une complète activation des lymphocytes B.

Hormones and Cell Regulation. N° 14, Eds J. Nunez, J.E. Dumont. Colloque INSERM/J. Libbey Eurotext Ltd. © 1989. Vol. 198, pp. 85-90

Towards an animal model for retinoblastoma

Rene Bernards*, Joan M. O'Brien**, Dennis M. Marcus**, Daniel M. Albert**, Tyler Jacks*** and Robert A. Weinberg***

* *Department of Molecular Genetics, The Cancer Center of the Massachussetts General Hospital and Harvard Medical School, Charlestown MA 02129 USA*
** *Howe Laboratory of Ophthalmology, Massachusetts Eye and Ear Infirmary, Harvard Medical School, Boston MA 02114 USA*
*** *Whitehead Institute for Biomedical Research and Department of Biology, Massachusetts Institute of Technology, Cambridge MA 02142 USA*

Within the past decade a large repertoire of cellular oncogenes has been implicated in the genesis of many types of cancers. These oncogenes all function to promote the neoplastic growth of cells in which they act. Indeed, they all appear to derive from normal cell genes, proto-oncogenes, which act to stimulate normal cell proliferation.

During this period, evidence has also been presented to suggest that elements that normally function to inhibit cell proliferation are also playing a role in the process of carcinogenesis. For instance, in a number of distinct types of tumors it was found that genetic material from specific chromosomal loci was absent in tumor DNAs, but present in the adjacent normal cell DNA. This indicates that loss of genetic material represents at least one step in the pathogenesis of these tumors (Klein, 1987). It seems likely that the normal function of the genes that are lost in these tumors is to restrain the growth of cells from which the tumors originate. For this reason such genes have been named recessive oncogenes or anti-oncogenes.

Retinoblastoma is an early childhood tumor occurring in about 1 out of every 20,000 live births and is probably the best-studied tumor in which loss of genetic material constitutes a critical step in tumorigenesis (reviewed by Klein et al., 1987; Friend et al., 1988; Hansen and Cavenee, 1988). Retinoblastoma occurs in two forms: An hereditary form in which an infant inherits one defective allele of the retinoblastoma (Rb) locus. The remaining wild-type allele is then lost relatively frequently through somatic mutation, resulting in a multifocal, bilateral form of retinoblastoma. The hereditary form of the disease constitutes about 30% to 40% of all cases. In the sporadic form, a new somatic mutation occurs in a retinal cell followed by the loss of the remaining normal allele through a second somatic event. The chance of spontaneous loss of both Rb alleles in a single cell is relatively low; as a consequence, non-hereditary retinoblastoma is unilateral and only a single focus of tumor growth is observed.

Another major difference between the familial and non-hereditary forms of retinoblastoma is that infants with familial retinoblastoma have only one functional copy of the Rb gene in all their somatic cells. The presence of only one functional allele of the Rb gene predisposes the patients with inherited retinoblastoma to a variety of tumors later in life, with osteosarcoma being the most frequently observed second tumor. In these second tumors, it was again found that the remaining functional Rb allele was lost in the tumor DNA, strongly implicating the loss of the Rb gene in the genesis of also these second tumors. These data furthermore suggest that the retinoblastoma gene plays a role in growth regulation of a much larger spectrum of tissues than just the retina.

Cytogenetic studies have shown that deletions in chromosome 13 region q14 are frequently found in the tumor genomes of retinoblastoma patients (Potluri et al., 1986). Recently we and others have isolated a cDNA clone from the q14 region of chromosome 13 that has many of the characteristics of the retinoblastoma gene (Friend et al. ,1986; Fung et al., 1987; Lee et al., 1987). Most importantly, Southern blot analysis of retinoblastoma tumor DNAs using the isolated cDNA as a probe revealed that as many as 30% of retinoblastomas have gross structural alterations in the locus that encodes this gene (Friend et al., 1986, 1987; Fung et al., 1987; Lee et al., 1987; Dunn et al., 1988; Goddard et al., 1988). Fine mapping of the deletions within this locus strongly suggested that the cDNA isolated indeed encodes the Rb gene.

Recently it has been shown that the Rb gene specifies a nuclear phosphoprotein of 105 kilodaltons (pp105 Rb) that binds to DNA in vitro (Lee et al., 1987; Whyte et al., 1988). Evidence that this gene product indeed mediates the growth suppressing effects of the intact Rb gene was recently provided by Huang et al. (1988), who showed that introduction of a retrovirus encoding pp105 Rb into a tumor cell line that lacks a functional Rb gene caused these tumor cells to become growth-arrested. Conversely it seems likely that the homozygous inactivation of this gene underlies the deregulated growth that initiates retinoblastoma.

In the past year, other studies have shown that the human Rb gene product is bound by the transforming proteins of adenovirus SV40 and human papilloma virus (DeCaprio et al., 1988; Whyte et al., 1988; Dyson et al., 1989). These data suggest that these tumor viruses acquire their oncogenic potential at least in part by complexing and inactivating the Rb gene product. Since these DNA tumor viruses have the ability to transform cells from a variety of tissues, it appears likely that the Rb gene product constitutes a critical regulator of growth in more cells than just the retina. Support for this view was also provided by recent observations made by several groups which investigated the status of the Rb gene in a number of tumors from patients that did not have a family history of retinoblastoma. They found homozygous inactivations of the Rb gene in such diverse tumors as breast cancer, small cell lung cancer, bladder cancer and a variety of mesenchymal tumors, again indicating the relevance of the Rb gene product in the normal growth control of breast, lung, bladder and mesenchymal tissues (Friend et al., 1987; Harbour et al., 1988; T'Ang et al., 1988; Horowitz et al., 1989).

The Rb gene is the first example of a gene whose inactivation leads to deregulated cell growth. The availability of a cloned copy of this gene should allow us to study the growth-inhibitory effect of its gene product in detail. One obstacle to the study of the function of the Rb gene is that to date no animal model for retinoblastoma exists. The reason for the apparent absence of retinoblastoma in domestic, agricultural and laboratory animals is at present unclear. For this reason, we have undertaken to develop an animal model for Rb-gene associated carcinogenesis, the first results of which are described here.

Structure and expression of the mouse Rb gene.

We recently isolated a nearly full length cDNA of the murine Rb gene. DNA sequence analysis of this clone revealed that the predicted structure of the murine Rb gene product has a 95% similarity to its human homologue (Bernards et al., 1989). Both the Rb protein of mouse and man were found to contain a leucine repeat motif (commonly referred to as a "leucine zipper") which is also found in the fos, myc and jun nuclear oncogenes, and appears to play a role in protein-protein interaction (Landschultz et al., 1988). The significance of the presence of this motif in the Rb protein is at present not clear.

To determine the pattern of expression of the mouse Rb gene, we have used Northern blot analysis of RNAs derived from mouse embryos at different periods of gestation. These data demonstrate that the Rb gene is expressed as early as 8 days of gestation, with a maximum level being observed at 14 days. When RNA derived from individual tissues of adult mice was tested for Rb expression we found that all tissues tested expressed the Rb gene, with brain, kidney, spleen, thymus and lung having relatively high levels and liver having relatively low levels of Rb mRNA (Bernards et al., 1989). These data again suggest that the Rb gene is involved in controlling cellular proliferation in a wide spectrum of cell types. On the other hand, these data raise the question why inactivation of the Rb gene leads to cancer in only a limited subset of tissues.

A mouse model for retinoblastoma.

We have recently been involved in the characterization of transgenic mice which harbor a transgene carrying the coding region of SV40 T-antigen oncogene coupled to the luteinizing hormone beta subunit gene promoter. Although one would expect that such transgenic mice would express the T-antigen gene in the cells of the anterior pituitary, a single founder mouse was found to develop bilateral ocular tumors. The retinal specificity of tumor formation was apparently caused by the fact that the SV40 T-antigen gene in this particular founder mouse was expressed only in the retina. Subsequent breeding of this founder mouse demonstrated that the ocular tumors were heritable and occurred with very high penetrance in offspring (Windle et.al., 1989).

One of the most striking histological characteristics of human retinoblastoma cells is that they spontaneously undergo photoreceptor cell differentiation in vivo to form Flexner-Wintersteiner rosettes. These rosettes are compsed of cuboidal cells which surround a central lumen. As can be seen in the photomicrograph in Fig. 1, rosettes that are very similar to those observed in human retinoblastoma were also found in every transgenic mouse ocular tumor examined. Furthermore, it was found that the transgenic mouse ocular tumors contained characteristic Homer Wright rosettes, retinoblastoma-characteristic ultrastructural features like lamelliform nuclear membranes, neurosecretory granules, cytoplasmic microtubules and cilia with a typical 9+0 pattern, thus lacking central tubules (Windle et al., 1989). All of these features are characteristic of human retinoblastoma, indicating that the ocular tumors observed in the transgenic mice closely resemble human retinoblastoma.

The mechanism by which ocular tumors arise in the transgenic mice is at present not clear. It seems likely that through a fortuitous integration the SV40 T-antigen gene was juxtaposed to a retinal-specific gene, bringing the transgene under the transcriptional control of this retinal-specific gene. Since SV40 T-antigen has been shown to bind to pp105 Rb (DeCaprio et al., 1988), it is likely that the expression of T-antigen in the retinal cells of the transgenic mice depletes these cells of functional Rb protein, thereby mimicking the loss of Rb by homozygous deletion.

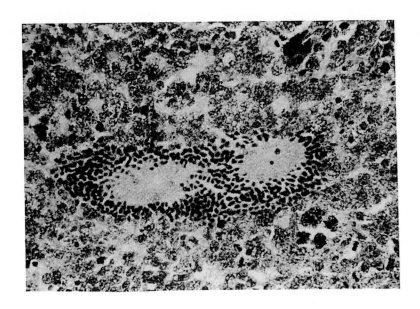

Figure 1. Photomicrograph of transgenic mouse ocular tumor section.
Shown are two differentiated Flexner-Wintersteiner rosettes composed of
photoreceptor-like cells, surrounded by more undifferentiated tumor cells.

Targeted mutagenesis.
Although the precise mechanism by which SV40 T-antigen induces ocular tumors in
this line of transgenic mice is not known, it is obvious that a tumor that is
by many criteria very similar to human retinoblastoma can be induced in mice.
Because of this, it is surprising that mice never seem to develop spontaneous
retinoblastoma. One possible explanation could be that not sufficient target
cells for oncogenic transformation are present in the mouse retina, making
retinoblastoma a very rare disease in mice. Alternatively it could be that loss
of Rb is associated with a different spectrum of tumors in mice than in humans,
or that Rb loss does not result in an increased risk for cancer in mice at all.

To answer these questions, we have begun experiments aimed at inactivating the
Rb gene in transgenic mice. One technique to achieve this goal, targeted
mutagenesis, was recently developed (See Capecchi, 1989 for a review). In
short, this technique involves the inactivation of one allele of Rb in mouse
embryo-derived stem cells (ES cells) in culture by homologous recombination,
followed by the introduction of these Rb+/Rb- cells in mouse blastocysts. The
resulting chimeric animals are then bred to derive mouse strains that are
hemizygous for Rb.

As a first step towards this goal, we have cloned a part of the genomic copy of
the mouse Rb gene that encodes exons 13 through 16. Using recombinant DNA
techniques, we have introduced several mutations in exon 16 of this clone of
the mouse Rb gene. The mutations consisted of either the insertion of a
stopcodon in the reading frame of the Rb coding sequence or the insertion of a
gene coding for neomycin resistance. These mutant Rb clones have been used for
either transfection or microinjection into mouse ES stem cells.

At present, we have identified by use of the PCR technique several pools of ES cells that contain cells that appear to have undergone at least one homologous recombination event. It should now be possible to isolate ES cells with only one functional copy of the Rb gene. Such cells, once isolated, should allow the generation of chimeric mice with only one functional copy of the Rb gene. The availability of these mice should allow us to ask whether loss of Rb leads to oncogenic transformation in mice and should also allow us to evaluate which additional factors (if any) are required to induce malignant transformation of murine cells in the absence of functional Rb protein.

References.

Bernards, R., Schackleford, G.M., Gerber, M.R., Horowitz, J.M., Friend, S.H., Schartl, M., Bogenmann, E., Rapaport, J.M., McGee, T., Dryja, T.P., and Weinberg, R.A. (1989): Structure and expression of the murine retinoblastoma gene and characterization of its encoded protein. Proc. Natl. Acad. Sci. USA. In press.

Capecchi, M,R. (1989): The new mouse genetics: altering the genome by gene targeting. Trends in Genetics 5: 70-76.

DeCaprio, J.A., Ludlow, J.W., Figge, J., Shew, J.Y., Huang, C.M., Lee, W.H., Marsilio, E., Paucha, E., and Livingston, D.M. (1988): SV40 large tumor antigen forms a specific complex with the product of the retinoblastoma susceptibility gene. Cell 54: 275-283.

Dunn, J.M., Phillips, R.A., Becker, A.J., and Gallie, B.L. (1988): Identification of germline ans somatic mutations affecting the retinoblastoma gene. Science 241: 1797-1800.

Dyson, N., Howley, P.M., Munger, K., and Harlow, E. (1989): The human papilloma virus 16 E7 oncoprotein is able to bind the retinoblastma gene product. Science 243: 934-936.

Friend, S.F., Bernards, R., Rogelj, S., Weinberg, R.A., Rapaport,J.M., Albert, D.M., and Dryja, T.P. (1986): A human DNA segment with properties of the gene that predisposes to retinoblastoma and osteosarcoma. Nature 323: 643-646.

Friend, S.H., Horowitz, J.M., Gerber, M.R., Wang, X.F., Bogenmann, E., Li, F.P., and Weinberg, R.A. (1987): Deletions of a DNA sequence in retinoblastomas and mesenchymal tumors: Organization of the sequence and its encoded protein. Proc. Natl. Acad. Sci. USA. 84: 9059-9063.

Friend, S.H., Dryja, T.P., and Weinberg, R.A. (1988): Oncogenes and tumor-suppressing genes. New England J. Med. 318: 618-622.

Fung, Y.T., Murphee, A.L., T'Ang, A., Qian, J., Hinrichs, S.H., and Benedict, W.F. (1987): Structural evidence for the authenticity of the human retinoblastoma gene. Science 236: 1657-1661.

Goddard, A.D., Balakier, H., Canton, M., Dunn, J., Squire, J., Reyes, E., Becker, A., Philips, R., and Gallie, B.L. (1988): Infrequent genomic rearrangement and normal expression of the putative RB1 gene in retinoblastoma tumors. Mol.Cell.Biol. 8: 2082-2088.

Hansen, M.F., and Cavenee, W.K. (1988): Retinoblastoma and the progression of tumor genetics. Trends in Genetics 4: 125-128.

Harbour, J.W., Lai, S.L., Whang-Peng, J., Gazdar, A.F., Minna, J.D., and Kaye, F.J. (1988): Abnormalities in structure and expression of the human retinoblastoma gene in SCLC. Science 241: 353-357.

Horowitz, J.M., Yandell, D.W., Park, S.H., Canning, S., Whyte, P., Buchkovich, K., Harlow, E., Weinberg, R.A., and Dryja, T.P. (1989): Point mutational inactivation of the retinoblastoma antioncogene. Science 243: 937-940.

Huang, H.J.S., Yee, J.K., Shew, J.Y., Chen, P.L., Bookstein, R., Friedmann, T., Lee, E.Y.H.P., and Lee, W.H. (1988): Suppression of the neoplastic phenotype by replacement of the RB gene in human cancer cells. Science 242: 1563-1566.

Klein, G. (1987): The approaching era of tumor suppressor genes. Science 238: 1539-1545.

Landschulz, W.H., Johnson, P.F., and McKnight, S.L. (1988): The leucine zipper: A hypothetical structure common to a new class of DNA binding proteins. Science 240: 1759-1763.

Lee, W.H., Shew, J.Y., Hong, F.D., Sery, T.W., Donoso, L., Young, J., Bookstein, R., and Lee, E.Y.H.P. (1987): The retinoblastoma susceptibility gene encodes a nuclear phosphoprotein associated with DNA binding activity. Nature 329: 642-645.

Potluri, V.R., Helson, L., Ellsworth, R.M., Reid, T., and Gilbert, F. (1986): Chromosmal abnormalities in human retinoblastoma. Cancer 58: 663-671.

T'Ang, A., Varley, J.M., Chakraborty, S., Murphee, A.L., and Fung, Y.K.T. (1988): Structural rearrangement of the retinoblastoma gene in human breast carcinoma. Science 242: 263-266.

Whyte, P., Buchkovich, K.J., Horowitz, J.M., Friend, S.H., Raybuck,M., Weinberg, R.A., and Harlow, E. (1988): Association between an oncogene and an anti-oncogene: the adenovirus E1A proteins bind the retinoblastoma gene product. Nature 334: 124-129.

Windle, J.J., Albert, D.M., O'Brien, J.M., and Mellon, P.L. (1989): Retinoblastoma in transgenic mice. Submitted for publication.

Hormones and Cell Regulation. N° 14, Eds J. Nunez, J.E. Dumont. Colloque INSERM/J. Libbey Eurotext Ltd. © 1989. Vol. 198, pp. 91-95

Transcriptional activity of the octamer motif in embryonic stem cells and preimplantation embryos

Hans R. Schöler, Rudi Balling, Antonis K. Hatzopoulos, Noriaki Suzuki and Peter Gruss

Max-Planck-Institute for Biophysical Chemistry, Department of Molecular Cell Biology, Am Faßberg, 3400 Göttingen, FRG

The molecular mechanisms that regulate mammalian embryogenesis are poorly understood. It is assumed that a network of regulatory genes controls the transformation of genetic information into embryonic structure. During the last years a number of mouse homeobox-containing genes were identified on the basis of sequence similarity to Drosophila genes (for review see Dressler and Gruss, 1988; Dressler, 1989; Serfling, 1989). Although it is assumed that their products are transcriptional regulatory proteins whose homeodomains interact with specific DNA sequences, their exact function and target sites still remain to be determined. Moreover, while the expression patterns (for ref. see Holland and Hogan, 1988) indicate a role in pattern formation, developmental activation of these genes is restricted to postimplantation stages of mouse development.

Sequence analysis of Oct1 and Oct2 cDNAs revealed the presence of a homeobox (for ref. see Schaffner, 1989). Oct1 and Oct2 are mammalian homeodomain-containing proteins whose target sequence is known but they are regarded to be ubiquitous and cell-specific transcription factors, respectively. We have analyzed various adult organs and different developmental stages of mouse embryos for the presence of octamer binding proteins. At least three new octamer binding proteins were identified in addition to the previously described Oct1 and Oct2 (Table 1). Oct1 is ubiquitously present in murine tissues, in agreement with cell culture data. Although Oct2 has been described as a B-cell specific protein, complexes of similar mobility to Oct2 were identified in the electrophoretic mobility shift assay (EMSA) using extracts from brain, kidney, embryo and sperm. However, despite their identical electrophoretic mobility they exhibit different binding properties. In embryo and brain at least one other protein, named Oct3, is present.

Table 1: Distribution of Oct1, Oct2, Oct3 and OC-C in different mouse tissues

	Ag8	liver	brain	kidney	12-day embryo	12-day placenta	12-day yolk
Oct1	+	+	+	+	+	+	+
Oct2/Oct2-like	+	-	+	+	+	-	-
Oct3/OC-C	+	-	+	-	+	-	-

Counting of days is according to Hogan et al. (1986). 12-day is 12.5 days p.c. (+/- 0.2). Ag8 is a IgG secreting mouse myeloma cell line.

A new microextraction procedure allowed the detection of two maternal octamer binding proteins, Oct4 and Oct5 (Table 2). Both proteins are present in unfertilized oocytes and embryonic stem cells. Additionally, Oct4 could be detected in primordial germ cells. However, Oct4 was not found in sperm or testis. Therefore Oct4 is present in cells of the female germline. Our results indicate that a family of octamer-binding proteins is present during mouse development and is differentially expressed during early embryogenesis. Since Oct4 and Oct5 are found in mouse oocytes these maternal proteins are prime candidates for regulatory factors active in preimplantation stages of mouse development. Protease clipping experiments of Oct4 and Oct1 suggest that both proteins contain similar DNA binding-domains.

The activity of the octamer motif was analyzed in two embryonic stem cell lines containing Oct4 and Oct5, the teratocarcinoma-derived EC cell line F9 and the blastocyst-derived ES cell line D3. It is known that oligomers of the octamer motif activate transcription in B-cells, where Oct2 is present (Gerster et al., 1987 and ref. therein). We demonstrate that the octamer motif can also strongly activate transcription in F9 and D3 stem cells which do not contain detectable levels of Oct2 but considerable amounts of Oct4 and Oct5. After differentiation of these cells, both the amount of Oct4 and Oct5 and the level of activation driven by the octamer motif are reduced. An intact octamer stimulates heterologous promoters in embryonic stem cells, whereas mutations in the octamer motif abolish transcriptional stimulation and binding of the octamer factors (Fig. 1).

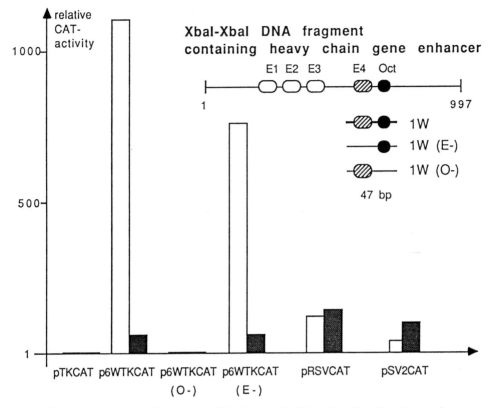

Fig. 1. Activity profile of the 6W enhancer in F9 cells. The F9 stem cells were differentiated 20 hrs after transfection. 68 hrs after transfection the undifferentiated (☐) and differentiated (■) F9 cells were harvested. pTKCAT contains a TK promoter in front of the CAT gene. p6WTKCAT: hexamer of the 1W fragment (Gerster et al., 1987) containing the E4 and the octamer motif of the heavy chain gene enhancer in front of the TK promoter. (O-): mutation in the octamer motif; (E-): mutation in the E4 motif (see diagram).

During the first stages of mouse development the blastomeres of the embryo are considered to be equipotent. Between the early eight-cell stage and the 16-cell stage the developmental potency of the cells becomes restricted. This results in the generation of two distinct lineages in the 16-cell morula: one or two internal cells give rise to the ICM, whereas most of the descendants of the external cells become trophectoderm. The trophectoderm develops into the extra-embryonic chorion, the outer portion of the placenta, whereas the ICM gives rise to the embryo.

Table 2: Germline specific expression of Oct proteins

	male PGCs	mature sperm	female PGCs	unfertilzed oocytes	mesonephros	D3/F9
Oct1	+	+	+	+	+	+
Oct2	-	+	-	-	-	-
Oct3	-	-	-	-	-	-
Oct4	+	-	+	+	-	+++
Oct5	-	-	-	+++	-	+

The isolation of the germ cells was carried out essentially as described by Hogan et al (1986). Genital ridges were dissected from the embryo around day 12.5 when the male and female genital ridges can be distinguished.

To study transcriptional actvity of the octamer motif in preimplantation embryos oligomers of the octamer motif and of a mutated octamer motif were microinjected in mouse oocytes. Interestingly, when the transgenic preimplantation embryos were analyzed the oligomerized octamer motif showed significant expression in the ICM but not in the trophoblast. Moreover, transcription seems to be restricted to certain cells of the ICM.

REFERENCES

Dressler, G.R. and Gruss, P. (1988): Do multigene families regulate
  vertebrate development? *Trends Genet.* **4**, 214-219

Dressler, G.R. (1989): An update on the vertebrate homeobox. *Trends Genet.* **5**,
  129-131.

Gerster, T., Matthias, P., Thali, M., Jiricny, J. and Schaffner, W. (1987): Cell
  type-specificity elements of the immunoglobulin heavy chain gene
  enhancer. *EMBO J.* **6**, 1323-1330.

Hogan, B.L.M., Constantini, F. and Lacy, E. (1986): *Manipulating the Mouse
  Embryo* (Cold Spring Harbor, New York: Cold Spring Harbor Laboratory)

Holland, P.W.H. and Hogan, B.L.M. (1988): Expression of homeo box genes during
  mouse development: A review. *Genes Dev.* **2**, 773-782.

Schaffner, W. (1989): How do different transcription factors binding the
  same DNA sequence sort out their jobs? TIG **5**, 37-39.

Serfling, E. (1989): Autoregulation - a common property of eukaryotic
  transcription factors? TIG **5**, 131-133.

Ion channels

Canaux ioniques

Hormones and Cell Regulation. N° 14, Eds J. Nunez, J.E. Dumont. Colloque INSERM/J. Libbey Eurotext Ltd. © 1989. Vol. 198, pp. 99-103

The role of the ATP-sensitive K-channel in stimulus-response coupling in the pancreatic ß-cell

S.J.H. Ashcroft and F.M. Ashcroft

Nuffield Department of Clinical Biochemistry, John Radcliffe Hospital, Headington, Oxford OX3 9DU and University Laboratory of Physiology, Parks Road, Oxford OX1 3PT, England

Introduction

Athough a number of hormones serve to increase plasma glucose levels, a reduction in blood glucose concentration is mediated almost entirely by insulin. Insulin therefore plays a key role in glucose homeostasis in man and higher mammals and a deficiency of insulin secretion leads to the severe metabolic disorders encountered in diabetes mellitus. There are two main types of diabetes. The most common form of diabetes, Type II or non-insulin dependent diabetes (NIDDM), may have a multifactorial aetiology but most often results from a failure of the ß-cell to release insulin in response to glucose stimulation. In patients with NIDDM, insulin secretion can however be stimulated by sulfonylureas such as glibenclamide which are used clinically in the treatment of this disorder.

There is considerable evidence, reviewed in [1], that the modulation of ionic channels plays a central role in stimulus-secretion coupling in the pancreatic ß-cell. All initiators of insulin secretion, including glucose and sulfonylureas, have the common property of depolarizing the ß-cell membrane and eliciting electrical activity [2]. Since it has been further established that glucose has to be metabolized by the ß-cell in order to stimulate both electrical activity [3] and insulin secretion [4], it is envisaged that an intracellular coupling factor mediates the effects of the sugar on electrical activity. We review here the evidence that the common denominator for effects of glucose metabolism and of sulfonylureas on ß-cell membrane electrical activity is a particular class of K-channel sensitive to intracellular ATP ($I_{K(ATP)}$). Such channels have been described in several cell types (for review see [5]) but their involvement in stimulus-secretion coupling appears unique to the ß-cell.

Electrical activity of the pancreatic ß-cell

Microelectrode recordings from intact islets have established that in the presence of a low concentration of glucose the ß-cell is electrically silent [6]. Raising the external glucose concentration to levels which stimulate insulin secretion produces an initial slow depolarisation of the ß-cell which brings the membrane to the threshold level at which electrical activity is initiated. It has long been known that this initial depolarisation results from a decrease in the membrane K-permeability [7]. The effect of glucose on the membrane potential (and K-permeability) is concentration dependent; low concentrations simply produce a dose-dependent depolarisation but do not elicit action potentials. At glucose concentrations above about 6mM, depolarisation is sufficient to open voltage-dependent Ca-channels and thereby elicit electrical activity. The increased influx of Ca^{2+} raises intracellular Ca^{2+} to levels sufficient to trigger exocytosis of insulin secretion granules.

In the ß-cell, electrical activity follows a characteristic pattern of slow oscillations in membrane potential (slow waves) on which the Ca-dependent action potentials are superimposed. Further increases in glucose concentration augment the frequency of these slow waves and action potentials. There is a good correlation between the frequency of action potentials, intracellular Ca^{2+} levels and insulin secretion.

Like glucose, sulfonylureas depolarize the ß-cell and initiate electrical activity [8].The molecular basis for these effects of glucose and of sulfonylureas on the ß-cell has been illuminated by recent patch-clamp studies on isolated single ß-cells.

Effects of glucose on $I_{K(ATP)}$

Cell-attached patch clamp studies [9] originally demonstrated that in the absence of glucose a single class of K-channel regulated the resting K-permeability of the ß-cell membrane; glucose caused a rapid, reversible and dose-dependent inhibition of channel activity. The ability of glucose to close the channels was abolished by metabolic inhibitors suggesting that glucose mediates its effect via an intracellular second messenger generated as a consequence of its metabolism. Other nutrient secretagogues, such as 2-ketoisocaproate, were also capable of blocking these channels [10].

Single channel currents show burst kinetics indicating at least two closed states, a short closed state represented by the brief closed state within the burst and a much longer closed state that determines the interburst interval [11]. The most marked effect of glucose is to decrease the duration of the bursts and cause the channel to remain in the long-lasting closed state for much longer, thereby reducing the probability of the channel being in the open state; the amplitude of the single channel current is unaltered [11]. The reduction in channel open probability is glucose-dependent and resembles that for the effect of glucose on membrane K-permeability; inhibition is half-maximal between 0 and 3mM glucose and almost complete by 7mM glucose. This supports the conclusion that the depolarization evoked by glucose is attributable to closing $I_{K(ATP)}$.

Effects of ATP on $I_{K(ATP)}$

Studies on excised inside-out patches revealed a K-channel with properties identical to that modulated by glucose metabolism which was inhibited by low concentrations of ATP applied to the cytosolic membrane surface [12,13]. The modulation of this channel by nucleotides has turned out to be complex. ATP has two distinct effects on channel activity. It inhibits $I_{K(ATP)}$ by a mechanism that does not involve protein phosphorylation and which is probably mediated by free ATP [14]. In addition MgATP, possibly via protein phosphorylation, is necessary to prevent and reverse the run-down of channel activity seen in excised membrane patches [15]. In inside-out patches the channel is extremely sensitive to inhibition by ATP with half maximal inhibition occurring at around 15 µM ATP [12,13,15]. In intact cells, however, the ATP sensitivity is apparently much less (see below). One possibility for this difference is that in the intact cell the inhibitory effect of ATP is reduced by ADP [16,17]. Effects of other nucleotides have also been described. In RINm5F ß-cells a stimulatory effect of GTP has been ascribed to activation of a GTP-binding protein [18].

ATP as a physiological regulator of $I_{K(ATP)}$

Several observations support a physiological role for ATP as a determinant of activity of $I_{K(ATP)}$. 1) Channel activity is blocked by ATP and no other relevant channel blockers have been identified. 2) In cell-attached patches, channel activity is increased by metabolic inhibitors which decrease cytosolic ATP levels and decreased by secretagogues which raise ATP levels. 3) There is a good correlation between the glucose-dependence of channel inhibition and that of the increase in ATP. 4) The time course of changes in intracellular ATP and in channel activity are similar. 5) The effects of glucose on channel kinetics resemble those of ATP. 6) Finally although it has been argued that there is a discrepancy between the ATP-sensitivity of the channel in the inside-out patch and the ATP concentration in the intact cell, this discrepancy is more apparent than real since the channel has a low open probability in the intact cell with more than 95% of channels closed in resting cells [19]. In addition the ATP-sensitivity in the inside-out patch appears much higher than that deduced from simultaneous measurements of ATP concentration and Rb-efflux in intact cells. This point was demonstrated in recent experiments in which we have studied the ATP-dependence of $I_{K(ATP)}$ in *intact* ß-cells of the cloned ß-cell line HIT-T15. $I_{K(ATP)}$ activity was measured as the glibenclamide-sensitive ^{86}Rb-efflux from preloaded HIT ß-cells and intracellular ATP was varied between 1-5mM by pre-exposure to varying concentrations of oligomycin. Marked activation of $I_{K(ATP)}$ was found when intracellular ATP was lowered below 3mM.

Possible reasons for the difference between the ATP sensitivity measured in the intact cell and the isolated patch include1) The ATP sensitivity in the inside-out patch is altered due to loss of additional channel modulators such as ADP. 2) ATP at the inner membrane surface may be lower than the measured total ATP for various reasons including sequestration by organelles; binding to diffusible macromolecules; cytosolic ATP gradients resulting from regional differences in ATP supply and utilization. 3) Removal of cytoskeletal connections on patch excision alters channel properties.

Effects of sulfonylureas on $I_{K(ATP)}$

Single channel recordings [20] have confirmed that in the ß-cell sulfonylureas act as specific blockers of $I_{K(ATP)}$.

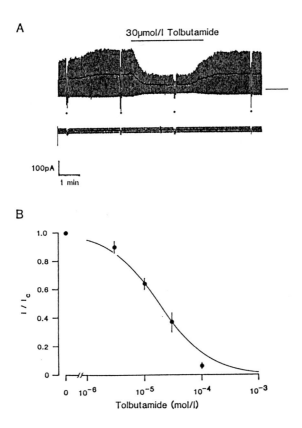

Figure 1. Effects of tolbutamide on whole-cell $I_{K(ATP)}$ -currents in a human ß-cell recorded as in [21] .

A. Whole cell currents (upper trace) and membrane potential (lower trace. The holding potential was -70mV and current responses to ±10mV pulses appear as vertical lines. The line on the right indicates the zero current potential and the asterisks indicate periods at which the holding potential was shifted to the zero current potential for measurement of the resting potential. 30μM tolbutamide was added to the bath for the period indicated by the horizontal line. B. Relationship between tolbutamide concentration and the whole cell current (I) expressed as a fraction of that in the absence of the drug (I_C).

Figure 1A shows inhibition of $I_{K(ATP)}$ measured in the whole cell patch clamp configuration by the sulfonylurea tolbutamide. The dose-response curve is shown in Figure 1B. The line is drawn to the Hill equation with a Hill coefficient of one indicating a one-to-one binding of the drug to the channel. Half-maximal inhibition is produced by 18μM tolbutamide which is similar to the concentration required to stimulate insulin release both in vitro and in vivo. This supports the view that the therapeutic action of sulfonylureas is a consequence of their ability to inhibit ATP-sensitive K-channels.

101

The sulfonylurea receptor

The high affinity of glibenclamide for the ATP-sensitive channel has provided a means for biochemical analysis of the sulfonylurea receptor. Equilibrium binding to membrane fractions from ß-cells has demonstrated saturable binding sites for sulfonylureas [22,23]. Several observations attest to the biological significance of the binding sites. The affinity of the binding sites correlates qualitatively and quantitatively with the ability of various sulfonylureas to elicit insulin release. The density of binding sites is sufficient to account for the number of channels estimated by patch clamp methods.

We have used [3H]glibenclamide to study the sulfonylurea receptor in membranes prepared from HIT-T15 ß-cells [24]. Scatchard plots of specific binding were curvilinear suggesting the possible presence of both high and low affinity sites and least squares regression analysis gave a better fit to a two-site than a single-site binding model with mean dissociation constants (n=5) of 1.12 ± 0.12 and 136 ± 23 nM for the high and low affinity sites. Both high and low affinity binding sites were present at around 5000 binding sites per cell. Since electrophysiological studies have shown that intracellular ADP modulates the ability of sulfonylurea to inhibit $I_{K(ATP)}$ [25] we investigated the interaction of ADP and other nucleotides with the [3H]glibenclamide binding-site. A marked reduction in binding was observed with physiological concentrations of ADP; ADP primarily reduced the apparent affinity of binding to the high affinity site with little effect on maximum binding suggesting that ADP may compete with glibenclamide. This effect was specific for ADP. When tested at a fixed (2nM) concentration of [3H]glibenclamide the following had no effect at 1mM: ATP, AMP, GTP, GDP, GMP, NADP, NADPH, NAD, NADH, guanosine, adenosine. Also without effect at 10μM were cAMP and cGMP. The sulfonamide diazoxide inhibits insulin release and has been shown electrophysiologically to cause opening of $I_{K(ATP)}$ [26]. However diazoxide, at a concentration (200μM) which markedly stimulates $I_{K(ATP)}$, had no effect on glibenclamide binding.

Radioactive glibenclamide has also been used as a probe for detection of the sulfonylurea binding-protein. Using [125I]glibenclamide we have detected binding activity on Western blots of HIT ß-cell membrane proteins after electrophoresis on non-denaturing gels [27]. In addition, [3H]glibenclamide has been used as a photoaffinity label; exposure to ultraviolet light of ß-cell tumour [28] or brain membranes [29] incubated with [3H]glibenclamide leads to covalent labelling of a protein of M_r 140-150kDal. Figure 2 demonstrates photoaffinity labelling of HIT-T15 ß-cell membranes with [3H]glibenclamide.

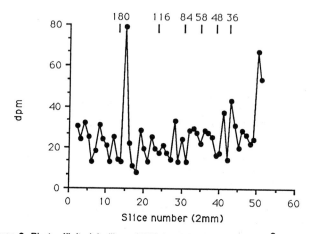

Figure 2. Photoaffinity labelling of HIT ß-cell membranes with [3H]glibenclamide.

Aliquots of HIT cell membrane proteins were incubated with 70nM [3H]glibenclamide (kindly supplied by Hoechst AG) for 1h in the dark. After exposure to ultraviolet light for 10 min proteins were precipitated and separated on a 7.5% SDS gel. Radioactivity was determined by liquid scintillation spectrometry after slicing the gel into 2mm pieces. The M_r's (kDal) of marker proteins are shown at the top of the figure.

After SDS gel electrophoresis, covalent incorporation of radioactivity into a polypeptide of M_r 150kDal can be observed. A 2500-fold purification of a glibenclamide-binding protein of similar M_r has been achieved from pig brain microsomes [29].

The close correlation between the affinity, specificity and density of sulfonylurea binding sites and the effects of sulfonylureas on $I_{K(ATP)}$ support the idea that the sulfonylurea receptor may constitute the $I_{K(ATP)}$ or a sub-unit of the channel. However it is still not possible to exclude the possibility that the sulfonylureas bind to a regulatory protein associated with the channel rather than to the channel itself. Functional reconstitution studies are required to resolve this point.

Relevance to NIDDM

There is good evidence, reviewed in [30], that NIDDM originates in a disorder of the ß-cell secretory machinery. Although we recognize that NIDDM may have multiple aetiology the ability of the diabetic ß-cell to respond to sulfonylureas suggests that events subsequent to the closing of $I_{K(ATP)}$ remain intact. The primary defect thus appears to be in the regulation of the $I_{K(ATP)}$. This may occur through a defective channel protein or as a consequence of altered glucose metabolism or impaired coupling of metabolism to channel activity. Studies on diabetic human ß-cells are needed to distinguish between these possibilities.

Acknowledgements

Studies from our laboratories have been supported by grants from the British Diabetic Association, the Medical Research Council, the EP Abraham Fund and Nordisk UK. FMA is a Royal Society 1983 University Research Fellow.

References

1. Henquin JC, Meissner HP (1984) Experientia 40: 1043-1052
2. Panten U (1987) ISI Atlas of Science: Pharmacology pp 307-310
3. Dean PM, Matthews EK, Sakamoto Y (1975) J Physiol 246: 459-478
4. Ashcroft SJH (1980) Diabetologia 18: 5-15
5. Ashcroft FM (1988) Ann Rev Neurosci 11: 97-118
6. Meissner HP (1976) J Physiol 72: 757-767
7. Henquin JC (1980) Biochem J 186: 541-550
8. Henquin JC, Meissner HP (1982) Biochem Pharmacol 31: 1407-1415
9. Ashcroft FM, Harrison DE, Ashcroft SJH (1984) Nature 312: 446-448
10. Ashcroft FM, Ashcroft SJH, Harrison DE (1987) J Physiol 385: 517-529
11. Ashcroft FM, Ashcroft SJH, Harrison DE (1987) J Physiol 400: 501-527
12. Rorsman P, Trube G (1985) Pflügers Arch 405: 305-309
13. Cook DL, Hales CN (1984) Nature 311: 271-273
14. Dunne MJ, Illot MC, Petersen OH (1987) J Membr Biol 99: 215-224
15. Ohno-Shosaku T, Zünkler BJ, Trube G (1987) Pflügers Arch 408: 133-138
16. Kakei M, Kelly RP, Ashcroft SJH, Ashcroft FM (1986) FEBS Lett 208: 63-66
17. Dunne MJ, Petersen OH (1986) FEBS Lett 208: 58-62
18. Dunne MJ, Petersen OH (1986) Pflügers Arch 407: 564-565
19. Cook DL, Satin LS, Ashford MLJ, Hales CN (1988) Diabetes 37: 495-498
20. Sturgess NC, Ashford MLJ, Cook DL, Hales CN (1986) Lancet ii: 474-475
21. Ashcroft FM, Kakei M, Gibson JS, Gray DW, Sutton R (1989) Diabetologia *In Press*
22. Gaines KL, Hamilton S, Boyd III AE (1988) J Biol Chem 263: 2589-2592
23. Schmid-Antomarchi H, De Weille J, Fosset M, Lazdunski M (1987) J Biol Chem 262: 15840-15844
24. Niki I, Kelly RP, Ashcroft SJH, Ashcroft FM (1989) Pflügers Arch *In Press*
25. Zünkler BJ, Lins S, Ohno-Shosaku T, Trube G, Panten U (1988) FEBS Lett 239: 241-244
26. Trube G, Rorsman P, Ohno-Shosaku T (1986) Pflügers Arch 407: 493-499
27. Ashcroft SJH, Hughes SJ, Kerr AJ (1988) Diabetologia 31: 466A
28. Kramer W, Oekonomopoulos R, Punter J, Summ H-D (1988) FEBS Lett 229: 355-359
29. Bernadi H, Fosset M, Lazdunski M (1988) Proc Natl Acad Sci 85: 9816-9820
30. Alford FP, Best JD (1984) In 'Recent Advances in Diabetes' Eds Nattrass M, Santiago JV. Churchill Livingstone

Hormones and Cell Regulation. N° 14, Eds J. Nunez, J.E. Dumont. Colloque INSERM/J. Libbey Eurotext Ltd. © 1989. Vol. 198, pp. 105-110

The plasma membrane Ca²⁺ pump : structural, functional and genetic aspects of isoform diversity

Emanuel E. Strehler, Roger Heim, Roland Fischer, Peter James, Thomas Vorherr, Gisela Vogel, Marie-Antoinette Strehler-Page and Ernesto Carafoli

Laboratory for Biochemistry, ETH Zurich, CH-8092 Zurich, Switzerland

INTRODUCTION

The precise control of intracellular free Ca^{2+} concentrations is a prerequisite for the function of Ca^{2+} as a second messenger in eukaryotic cells. Ca^{2+} pumps of cell membranes play a crucial role in the maintenance and fine-tuning of the intracellular Ca^{2+} concentrations (Pedersen & Carafoli, 1987; Carafoli, 1987). They belong to the class of P-type ion transport ATPases (Schatzmann, 1982; Penniston, 1983; Pedersen & Carafoli, 1987) among which they are distinguished by their high molecular weight of approximately 140 kDa and by their interaction with, and direct stimulation by, Ca^{2+}-calmodulin (Penniston, 1983; Carafoli, 1987). Ca^{2+} pumps have been detected, with essentially the same general properties, in all plasma membranes examined (the liver enzyme, however, appears to differ significantly in some properties such as calmodulin affinity and molecular weight (F. Kessler, F. Bennardini and E. Carafoli, unpublished observations)), but recent work involving direct peptide sequencing and molecular cloning methods indicates that distinct isoforms exist for this pump which may differ in some of their properties (Shull & Greeb, 1988; Verma et al., 1988; Strehler et al., submitted). In this report we will concentrate on the recent progress made in our Laboratory on the elucidation of the primary structure and mechanism of generation of various Ca^{2+} pump isoforms, and on the possible arrangement of some functional and regulatory domains in this enzyme.

PRIMARY STRUCTURE OF TWO CALCIUM PUMP ISOFORMS AND ASSIGNMENT OF MAJOR DOMAINS

The first complete primary structure of a human plasma membrane Ca^{2+} pump as deduced from its cloned cDNA has been reported by Verma et al. (1988), while the amino acid sequences of two isoforms of the rat Ca^{2+} pump have been determined independently by Shull & Greeb (1988). Recently, the primary structure of a novel, second human Ca^{2+} pump isoform has been determined by molecular cloning methods (Strehler et al., submitted). Whereas the first human Ca^{2+} pump isoform is clearly related to the rat protein PMCA1 (Shull & Greeb, 1988) the novel human pump isoform does not correspond to the rat isoform PMCA2 but rather represents a third type of Ca^{2+} pump. The primary structures of the two human plasma membrane Ca^{2+} pump isoforms are displayed in Fig. 1. The cDNA clones coding for the first isoform (tera) were isolated from a teratoma cell library while those specifying the second isoform (int) were originally isolated from a small intestinal mucosa library. The two proteins consist of 1,220 and 1,205 amino acid residues with calculated molecular weights of 134,683 and 133,930, respectively.

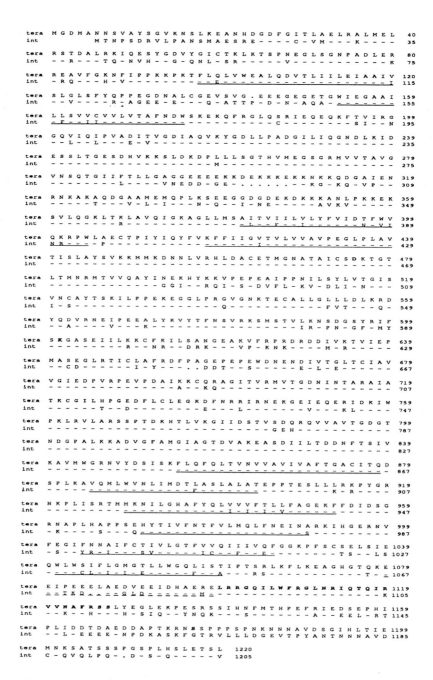

Fig. 1. Amino acid sequences of two human plasma membrane Ca^{2+} pumps and identification of major domains. The cDNA-deduced sequences of a human "teratoma" (tera) and an "intestinal mucosa" (int) isoform have been aligned. Dashes indicate sequence identity, dots indicate deletions introduced to optimize the alignment. The ten putative transmembrane domains are underlined, the important residues Asp-475, Lys-601 and Ser-1178 as well as the calmodulin binding region of the "tera" sequence are printed in boldface. The putative Ca^{2+} binding region is underlined with a dashed line.

Independent determinations of peptide sequences obtained after specific modification and cleavage procedures on the purified erythrocyte protein, as well as sequence comparisons with known P-type ion-pumps such as the Ca^{2+} ATPases of sarcoplasmic reticulum (Brandl et al., 1986), the α-subunits of Na^+/K^+ ATPases (Shull et al., 1986) and the H^+/K^+ ATPases (Shull & Lingrel, 1986) have led to the identification of a number of important functional domains along the primary sequence of this pump (Filoteo et al., 1987; James et al., 1988, 1989; Verma et al., 1988; Carafoli et al., 1989). In Fig. 1 residues and domains of critical importance to the Ca^{2+} ATPase function and structure are indicated: The site of aspartyl phosphate formation (Asp-475 and Asp-465 in the two isoforms, respectively), the lysine residue (Lys-601/Lys-591) which binds the ATP analog FITC, the calmodulin binding region (residues 1100 to 1127/1087 to 1113) as well as the ten hydrophobic regions suggested by the Kyte-Doolittle algorithm (Kyte & Doolittle, 1982) as putative transmembrane domains.

Immediately N-terminal to the calmodulin binding domain a stretch of negatively charged amino acids (underlined with a dashed line in Fig. 1) could presumably be involved in Ca^{2+} binding: In the absence of calmodulin it would not be free to bind Ca^{2+}; instead, the adjoining calmodulin binding region would interact with the acidic putative Ca^{2+} binding region. Binding of calmodulin could induce a conformational change, swinging the positively charged calmodulin binding region away from the acidic putative Ca^{2+} binding site, thus freeing the latter to bind Ca^{2+} (Carafoli et al., 1989). Work in our Laboratory with synthetic peptides has provided some experimental support for this model: The synthetic basic calmodulin binding domain interacts with calmodulin in a Ca^{2+} dependent manner, and the putative Ca^{2+} binding domain interacts very strongly with the basic calmodulin binding domain in the absence of Ca^{2+} (Vorherr et al., submitted).

The C-terminal regulatory region of the Ca^{2+} pump contains a further region of interest: It has been shown previously that the Ca^{2+} dependent ATPase activity of the erythrocyte Ca^{2+} pump can be stimulated by phosphorylation via the cAMP dependent protein kinase (Caroni & Carafoli, 1981; Neyses et al., 1985; James et al., 1989). Direct sequencing of the erythrocyte pump peptide labeled upon phosphorylation by the cAMP kinase has resulted in the identification of a serine residue as the phosphorylation target (James et al., 1989) which is embedded in a sequence that matches only to the "teratoma" sequence (Ser-1178 in Fig. 1). The C-terminal sequences are highly divergent in the two pump isoforms, and since this region appears to be crucially involved in the regulation of Ca^{2+} pump function its careful analysis is of particular interest.

CALCIUM PUMP ISOFORMS ARE GENERATED FROM A MULTIGENE FAMILY AND BY ALTERNATIVE RNA PROCESSING

The two human isoforms displayed in Fig. 1 share 75% sequence identity (88% similarity using the "Bestfit" program of the UWCGC software). The distribution of amino acid (and nucleotide) sequence differences between the two human isoforms along the entire length of the molecules indicates that they are the products of separate genes. The same is true for the two rat Ca^{2+} pump isoforms PMCA1 and PMCA2 which are also separate gene products (Shull & Greeb, 1988). As mentioned earlier, rat PMCA1 corresponds to the human "tera" isoform whereas rat PMCA2 is distinct from the human "int" protein. cDNA clones coding for the human equivalent of the rat PMCA2 isoform have recently also been isolated in our Laboratory (R. Heim, R. Fischer, and E. Strehler, unpublished results), indicating that the human plasma membrane Ca^{2+} pump gene family consists of at least three separate members. The recently published partial sequence of a bovine Ca^{2+} pump (Brandt et al., 1988) is sufficiently divergent from the three isoforms mentioned above to suggest that the actual number of genes encoding mammalian plasma membrane Ca^{2+} pump isoforms may even be higher. Preliminary evidence shows that at least some of these genes map to different chromosomes in the human genome (W. McBride, S. Olson, E. Strehler, and E. Carafoli, unpublished observations). Almost nothing is presently known, however, about the tissue distribution of the various pump isoforms and about the possible regulatory mechanisms controlling Ca^{2+} pump gene expression.

Further plasma membrane Ca^{2+} pump isoform diversity may be generated by alternative RNA splicing. cDNA clones have been isolated from a human fetal skeletal muscle library that are identical to those encoding the "teratoma" Ca^{2+} pump except for an "insertion" of either 87 bp or 114 bp between amino acid codons 1117 and 1118. These insertions encode 29 and 38 residues and, if expressed as protein, would lead to Ca^{2+} pump isoforms containing 1249 and 1258 residues, respectively (Strehler et al., submitted). Perhaps significantly, these insertions occur precisely within the calmodulin binding region of the pump (see below). A genomic clone covering the region of interest in these cDNAs has been isolated and characterized (Strehler et al., submitted): Analysis of the exon-intron structure showed that the 87 and 114 bp "insertions" are encoded within a separate 154 bp exon that can be differentially processed to generate four mature mRNAs (Fig. 2a). Sequence comparison shows that the cDNA coding for the rat PMCA1 Ca^{2+} pump isoform (Shull & Greeb, 1988) is, in fact, generated from an mRNA that contains the complete 154 bp "alternative" exon. Since the 154 bp insertion leads to a shift in the reading rame and to a stop codon after residue 1176, this Ca^{2+} pump is considerably shorter at its C-terminus than the other, closely related, isoforms.

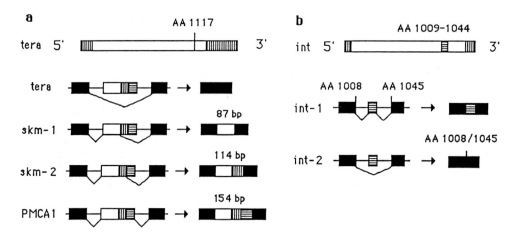

Fig. 2. Alternative RNA splicing as a mechanism to generate Ca^{2+} pump isoform diversity.
a: Top, scheme of the "teratoma" pump cDNA. 5' and 3' untranslated sequences are stippled, the position after codon 1117 where alternative splicing leads to different mRNAs is indicated. Bottom, differential splicing pathways involving a single exon of the "teratoma" Ca^{2+} pump gene.
b: Top, scheme of the "intestinal mucosa" pump cDNA. The area involved in alternative RNA processing (codons 1009 to 1044) is indicated. Bottom, splicing pathways leading to int-1 and int-2 mRNAs. See text for more details.

Alternative RNA processing may also be involved in the generation of Ca^{2+} pump isoforms of the human "intestinal mucosa" type (Fig. 2b). A cDNA clone has been isolated which is identical to those coding for the second ("int") human pump isoform except that it lacks 108 bp corresponding to amino acid codons 1009 to 1044 of the sequence shown in Fig.1 (R. Heim, R. Fischer, and E. Strehler, unpublished results). Interestingly, these 108 bp are precisely specified by a single exon in the "teratoma" Ca^{2+} pump gene (M.-A. Strehler-Page, personal communication), strongly indicating that alternative exon splicing may also be involved in the generation of mRNA species coding for isoforms of the second human Ca^{2+} pump. The question of whether the various isoforms that could theoretically be generated from the differentially processed mRNAs are indeed expressed in vivo is of interest because these proteins would vary in some important domains suggesing possible differences in their structure, function and regulation (see below).

As might be expected, several domains of known functional importance are highly cvonserved in the different plasma membrane Ca^{2+} pump isoforms (Fig.1). These include the region encompassing the site of acylphosphate formation, the FITC (ATP-) binding site as well as other regions previously shown to be conserved among ion-transporting ATPases (Verma et al., 1988; Fischer, 1989). To test existing models of the structure, function and regulation of the plasma membrane Ca^{2+} pump the regions of sequence divergence among different isoforms are of particular interest. For example, proof of the existence and of a normal function of a Ca^{2+} pump generated from the alternatively spliced mRNA lacking the exon coding for amino acids 1009 to 1044 of the "intestinal mucosa" pump (int-2 in Fig. 2b) would force us to re-evaluate the model proposing ten membrane spanning regions in this molecule. In the sequence shown in Fig.1 "deletion" of residues 1009 to 1044 would remove transmembrane domain 10, leading to a product with an odd number of transmembrane domains. Since the C-terminal regulatory region and the part of the protein that contains the catalytic (ATP binding) domain must both be located intracellularly, the number of membrane spanning domains between these two regions must be even. This would mean, then, that one of the 5 remaining hydrophobic stretches in the C-terminal half of the molecule would actually not be traversing the membrane in vivo. Detailed studies with specific antibodies raised against selected peptide sequences may help to solve this problem.

The differences in the C-terminal regulatory region of isoforms generated from alternatively spliced mRNAs of the "teratoma" type (Fig. 2a) are also of interest. The "insertion" of amino acids - due to the inclusion of additional exon sequences in the corresponding mRNAs - occurs precisely within the calmodulin binding domain of the Ca^{2+} pump. Although 6 out of the 10 first residues of the "insertion" sequence (Fig. 3) are identical to the sequence of residues 1118 to 1127 as shown in Fig. 1, these "insertions" might well affect the calmodulin regulation of the enzyme. Replacement of the basic residues Arg-1119 and Arg-1125 by Asp and Gln, respectively, could be of consequence because calmodulin binding domains generally exhibit a strongly basic character assumed to be important for their interaction with calmodulin (James et al., 1988).

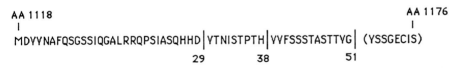

AA 1118

MDVYNAFQSGSSIQGALRRQPSIASQHHD|YTNISTPTH|VVFSSSTASTTVG| (YSSGECIS)

AA 1176

29   38   51

Fig. 3: Sequence of the "insertion" region encoded by the 154 bp alternatively spliced exon of the "teratoma" Ca^{2+} pump gene. Depending on the splicing pathway 29, 38 or 51 amino acids are inserted after residue 1117. In the last case, a shift in reading frame leads to an altered and considerably shorter C-terminal sequence (indicated in brackets).

Further regions of striking sequence divergence are located at the extreme termini (Fig. 1). While the significance of N-terminal sequence variation among Ca^{2+} pump isoforms is not clear at present, the C-terminal region after the calmodulin binding domain appears to be involved in the regulation of the enzyme (Verma et al., 1988; Carafoli et al., 1989). While phosphorylation by the cAMP dependent kinase has been shown to occur at Ser-1178 of the "teratoma" Ca^{2+} pump (James et al., 1988), no canonical sequence for phosphorylation by this kinase is present in the corresponding region of the "intestinal mucosa" isoform and of the Ca^{2+} pump generated from a "teratoma-type" mRNA containing the complete 154 bp alternatively spliced exon. These findings indicate that different pump isoforms may show differences in their mode of regulation. Final proof of the suggested functional, structural and regulatory differences between plasma membrane Ca^{2+} pump isoforms is crucially dependent on studies of the purified proteins. Expression of each isoform from its corresponding cDNA, combined with site-directed mutagenesis to alter specific residues, promise to shed more light on these questions in the near future.

ACKNOWLEDGEMENTS

The original work described in this contribution was supported by the Swiss National Science Foundation (grant 3.531-0-86).

REFERENCES

Brandl, C.J., Green, N.M., Korczak, B. & MacLennan, D.H. (1986): Two Ca^{2+} ATPase genes: Homologies and mechanistic implications of deduced amino acid sequences. *Cell* 44, 597-607.

Brandt, P., Zurini, M., Neve, R.L., Rhoads, R.E. & Vanaman, T.C. (1988): A C-terminal, calmodulin-like regulatory domain from the plasma membrane Ca^{2+}-pumping ATPase. *Proc. Natl. Acad. Sci. U.S.A.* 85, 2914-2918.

Carafoli, E. (1987): Intracellular calcium homeostasis. *Annu. Rev. Biochem.* 56, 395-433.

Carafoli, E., James, P., Strehler, E. & Penniston, J.T. (1989): The calcium pump of the plasma membrane: structure-function relationships. In: *Proceedings of the 6th International Symposium on Calcium Binding Proteins in Health and Disease*, ed. H. Hidaka. New York: Plenum Publishing Corp., in press.

Caroni, P. & Carafoli, E. (1981): Regulation of Ca^{2+}-pumping ATPase of heart sarcolemma by a phosphorylation-dephosphorylation process. *J. Biol. Chem.* 256, 9371-9373.

Filoteo, A.G., Gorski, J.P. & Penniston, J.T. (1987): The ATP-binding site of the erythrocyte membrane Ca^{2+} pump. *J. Biol. Chem.* 262, 6526-6530.

Fischer, R. (1989): Molecular cloning of a human plasma membrane Ca^{2+}-ATPase. Ph.D. thesis no. 8811, ETH Zurich.

James, P., Maeda, M., Fischer, R., Verma, A.K., Krebs, J., Penniston, J.T. & Carafoli, E. (1988): Identification and primary structure of a calmodulin binding domain of the Ca^{2+} pump of human erythrocytes. *J. Biol. Chem.* 263, 2905-2910.

James, P.H., Pruschy, M., Vorherr, T.E., Penniston, J.T. & Carafoli, E. (1989): Primary structure of the cAMP-dependent phosphorylation site of the plasma membrane calcium pump. *Biochemistry*, in press.

Kyte, J. & Doolittle, R.F. (1982): A single method for displaying the hydropathic character of a protein. *J. Mol. Biol.* 157, 105-132.

Neyses, L., Reinlib, L. & Carafoli, E. (1985): Phosphorylation of the Ca^{2+} pumping ATPase of heart sarcolemma and erythrocyte plasma membrane by the cAMP-dependent protein kinase. *J. Biol. Chem.* 260, 10283-10287.

Pedersen, P.L. & Carafoli, E. (1987): Ion-motive ATPases. *Trends Biochem. Sci.* 12, 146-150 and 186-189.

Penniston, J.T. (1983): Plasma membrane Ca^{2+}-ATPases as active Ca^{2+} pumps. In *Calcium and Cell function*, ed. W.Y Cheung, Vol. IV, pp. 99-149. New York: Academic Press.

Schatzmann, H.J. (1982): The calcium pump of erythrocytes and other animal cells. In *Membrane Transport of Calcium*, ed. E. Carafoli, pp. 41-108. London: Academic Press.

Shull, G.E. & Greeb, J. (1988): Molecular cloning of two isoforms of the plasma membrane Ca^{2+}-transporting ATPase from rat brain. *J. Biol. Chem.* 263, 8646-8657.

Shull, G.E. & Lingrel, J.B. (1986): Molecular cloning of the rat stomach $(H^+ + K^+)$ ATPase. *J. Biol. Chem.* 261, 16788-16791.

Shull, G.E., Greeb, J. & Lingrel, J.B. (1986): Molecular cloning of three distinct forms of the Na^+,K^+-ATPase α-subunit from rat brain. *Biochemistry* 25, 8125-8132.

Verma, A.K., Filoteo, A.G., Stanford, D.R., Wieben, E.D., Penniston, J.T., Strehler, E.E., Fischer, R., Heim, R., Vogel, G., Mathews, S., Strehler-Page, M.-A., James, P., Vorherr, T., Krebs, J. & Carafoli, E. (1988): Complete primary structure of a human plasma membrane Ca^{2+} pump. *J. Biol. Chem.* 263, 14152-14159.

Hormones and Cell Regulation. N° 14, Eds J. Nunez, J.E. Dumont. Colloque INSERM/J. Libbey Eurotext Ltd. © 1989. Vol. 198, pp. 111-116

Growth control by proton transport : evolutionary considerations and novel approaches based on the cloned yeast proton pump

Ramon Serrano* and Rosario Perona**

* European Molecular Biology Laboratory, Meyerhoffstrasse 1, 6900 Heidelberg, Germany
** Instituto de Investigaciones Biomedicas del CSIC, Arzobispo Morcillo 4, 28029 Madrid, Spain

INTRODUCTION

Despite intensive efforts during the last years, the growth control circuits of eukaryotic cells have yet to be elucidated. The on going discovery of oncogenes, transcription factors, G-proteins and protein kinases is advancing our knowledge at the descriptive level, but not in terms of understanding (Maddox, 1988). Although there is hope that further description will uncover mechanisms, the present state of the field of growth control is one of scientific crisis. This is not because an old paradigm is under question (Kuhn, 1970) but because of a lack of models which could illuminate and help order the collected data.

We wish to re-explore an early hypothesis of growth control by proton transport (Loeb, 1913) and to outline a new defense of it based on evolutionary considerations and on some novel experimental approaches which employ the cloned yeast proton pump.

EVOLUTION OF PROTON TRANSPORT

The origin of proton pumps can be traced back to the requirements for intracellular pH regulation in primitive cells (Raven and Smith, 1976). Acids generated by fermentation were detrimental to intracellular enzymes and cells developing proton pumps driven by either ATP, redox processes or light had a selective advantage. Later on proton transport assumed other physiological functions such as the regulation of cell volume mediated by a

H+/Na+ antiport and the active transport of nutrients mediated by H+-symports (Wilson and Lin, 1980).

Two types of H+-ATPases evolved independently: (1) the complex (F_0F_1) H+-ATPases found in bacteria and the eukaryotic organelles which probably derived from them (mitochondria, chloroplasts and vacuoles; Nelson and Taiz, 1989) and (2) the simple (E-P) H+-ATPases of the plasma membrane of plants, fungi and protozoa (Serrano, 1988). The combination in the same bacterial cell of (F_0F_1) H+-ATPases and other proton pumps driven by either redox reactions or light provide the basis for oxidative and photosynthetic phosphorylations (Raven and Smith, 1976). (F_0F_1) H+-ATPases were therefore converted into "coupling factors", working under physiological conditions in the direction of ATP synthesis. The (E-P) H+-ATPases of eukaryotic cells, however, followed a different evolutionary pathway and diversified into enzymes pumping Na+, K+ and Ca^{2+} (Serrano, 1988).

The two main lineages of eukaryotic cells also differ in the type of cation pumping (E-P) ATPase found in their plasma membrane. In plant cells that evolved in fresh water, the primitive H+-ATPase is preserved, nutrient uptake occurs by H+-symport and the regulation of cell volume is mostly achieved by the presence of a rigid cell wall. Animal cells specialized for life in the Na+-rich medium of sea water, did not not develop a rigid cell wall and utilize the extrusion of Na+ by a Na+,K+-ATPase for volume regulation (Tosteson, 1964). Animal cells changed the cation specificity of active cotransport systems to develop Na+-symports and utilize the primitive H+/Na+ antiport for proton efflux instead of Na+ efflux, as in bacteria and plant cells.

EVOLUTION OF GROWTH CONTROL

In primitive cells growth control was solely based on substrate availability for the different enzymes. When substrates were lacking the cell division cycle would be interrupted. This is detrimental because in this interrupted state the cells are more susceptible to damage. A "premonition" control device evolved such that cells commit to a division cycle by anticipating substrate sufficiency for all the required enzymes. This type of control is observed in present day microorganisms, such as yeast, where the nutritional state controls the "start" step of the cell cycle (Pringle and Hartwell, 1981). Multicellular organisms need more sophisticated controls superimposed on nutritional constraints. These are based on growth factors produced by other cells according to a developmental programme and which integrate the growth of individual cells with the needs of the whole organism.

Regulation of proton transport could have provided the basic mechanism for primitive growth control. In yeast (Gillies et al., 1981) and in *Dictyostelium* (Aerts et al., 1985) there is an increase in intracellular pH at the beginning of the cell cycle and this is probably due to activation of plasma membrane H+-ATPase. A mutational analysis has demonstrated that the yeast plasma membrane H+-ATPase is both essential and rate limiting for growth. (Serrano, 1988). In addition to driving active nutrient transport, the ATPase generates a high intracellular pH. This may transmit a general growth signal to the many enzymatic machineries involved in growth and which operate best at high pH. These include the ribosomes and the RNA polymerase and DNA polymerase complexes. The utilization of pH as intracellular signal offers several advantages, including pleiotropic effects on many different enzymes and a connection with the bioenergetic state of the plasma membrane, assuring a coupling between nutrient uptake and biosynthetic metabolism.

In higher plants growth promoting factors such as the auxin hormones and the phytotoxin fusicoccin activate the plasma membrane proton pump. Although intracellular alkalinization is also probably important, plant physiologist have primarily considered the resulting extracellular acidification, which somehow triggers the loosening of the cell wall and allows expansive growth driven by turgor (Marre, 1979). In animal cells growth promoting factors activate the H+/Na+ antiporter and increase intracellular pH (Epel and Dube, 1987). Therefore, the primitive signaling system based on modulation of proton transport is retained in higher organisms. This is true even in animal cells, where the major chemiosmotic circuit at the plasma membrane is no longer based on protons.

THE COMPLEXITY OF THE EARLY GROWTH RESPONSE OF HIGHER EUKARYOTES

When quiescent cells of animals (Baserga and Surmacz, 1987) or plants (Guilfoyle, 1986) are induced to grow by the addition of growth factors there is a complex early response where ,in addition to the activation of proton transport, the cells activate different protein kinases and induce the transcription of many genes. It is difficult to ascertain the extent many of these early responses actually represent biosynthetic processes or correspond to regulatory mechanisms operating at the beginning of the cell cycle. It is unlikely that so many different phenomena relate to the modulation of proton transport and therefore alternative regulatory pathways should operate. These pathways include protein kinase cascades (Hunter, 1987) and may have evolved to complement and interdigitate with the primitive regulatory circuit based on proton transport.

Questions arise about the order of events in this regulatory circuit. There is a major controversy about the role of the proton transport response (Grinstein et al., 1989). The interpretation that it is only a permissive factor for other processes may be related to its ancient role as a general trigger for growth as discussed above. It is possible that in present day organisms protein kinases are the important pace-makers of the cell cycle and that proton transport plays only a secondary role. However, several examples indicate that a trigger role for proton transport cannot be fully discarded. Chemically mutagenized fibroblasts, which become tumorigenic, exhibit an increased intracellular pH due to altered properties of H^+/Na^+ exchange (Ober and Pardee, 1987). Alkaline pH has a mitogenic effect (Zetterberg and Engstrom, 1981), expression of oncogenes causes intracellular alkalinisation (Doppler et al., 1987) and this is the signal which best correlates with cell growth (Hesketh et al., 1988). Finally, in vivo measurements of tumors with ^{31}P NMR indicates an elevation of intracellular pH (Oberhaensli et al., 1986) and a high microenvironmental pH may have a role in the etiology of epithelial human cancer (Harguindey et al., 1989).

The main argument against a role of intracellular pH as a mediator of the growth response is that the presence of high bicarbonate concentrations maintains a high intracellular pH in animal cells even in the absence of growth factors (Thomas, 1989; Grinstein et al., 1989). However, it seems that this "buffering" effect of bicarbonate is concentration dependent and it is not clear if the physiological levels prevailing in the tissues (much lower than in the blood) can abolish pH changes during the growth response.

TRANSFORMATION WITH HETEROLOGOUS PROTON PUMP GENES

The major experimental problem in evaluating the effect of intracellular pH changes on the growth response is that alkaline media or ammonia, utilized in the past for this purpose, have toxic effects. What is needed are means to specifically manipulate intracellular pH without affecting either external pH or the pH of internal acidic organelles (lysosomes, vacuoles, secretory pathway, endosomes). We have approached this problem by introducing and expressing in heterologous cells the gene for the yeast plasma membrane H^+-ATPase under control of adequate promoters (Perona and Serrano, 1988). In the case of monkey and mouse fibroblasts, a tumorigenic transformation occurred, which correlates with increased intracellular pH. Controls, with inactive mutants of the yeast ATPase obtained by site-directed mutagenesis, did not transform the same fibroblasts. More recent data indicate that cells expressing the yeast H^+-ATPase are electrically hyperpolarized, as expected from the strong electrogenic character of the yeast enzyme (Serrano, 1988). In addition, as expected from the acid-extrusion capability of the enzyme, these fibroblasts can survive a H^+-suicide selection (Pouysegur et al., 1984) which kills normal cells. We are now extending these observations to other H^+-ATPases genes and are characterizing the state in these cells of other regulatory signals, such as protein kinases, transcription factors etc. Now that intracellular pH has been specifically manipulated and cell growth promoted, this experimental system could allow a dissection of the early growth response and the identification of the steps bypassed by the pH signal.

REFERENCES

Aerts, R. J., Durston, A. J. and Moolenaar, W. H. (1985): Cytoplasmic pH and the regulation of the Dictyostelium cell cycle. *Cell* 43, 653-657.

Baserga, R. and E. Surmacz (1987): Oncogenes, cell cycle genes and the control of cell proliferation. *Bio/Technology* 5, 355-358.

Doppler, W., Jaggi, R. and Groner, B. (1987): Induction of v-mos and activated Ha-ras oncogene expression in quiescent NIH 3T3 cells causes intracellular alkalinisation and cell cyle progression. *Gene* 54, 147-153.

Epel, D. and Dube, F. (1987): Intracellular pH and cell proliferation. In *Control of Animal Cell Proliferation*. Vol. II. Eds. A. L. Boynton and H. L. Leffert, pp.363-393. New York: Academic Press.

Gillies, R. J., Ugurbil, K., Den Hollander, J. A. and Shullman, R. G. (1981): ^{31}P NMR studies of intracellular pH and phosphate metabolism during cell division cycle of *Saccharomyces cerevisiae*. *Proc. Natl. Acad. Sci. USA* 78, 2125-2129.

Grinstein, S., D. Rotin and M. J. Mason (1989): Na^+/H^+ exchange and growth factor-induced cytosolic pH changes. Role in cellular proliferation. *Biochim. Biophys. Acta* 988, 73-97.

Guilfoyle, T. J. (1986): Auxin-regulated gene expression in higher plants. *CRC Critical Rev. Plant Sci.* 4, 247-276.

Harguindeay, S., L. M. A. Aparicio and S. M. Algarra (1989): Integrated etiopathogenesis of cancer of mucosal surfaces with emphasis on the digestive tract: an appraisal. *J. Biol. Response Modifiers* 8, 1-10.

Hesketh, T. R., Morris, J. D. H., Moore, J. P. & Metcalfe, J. C. (1988): Ca^{2+} and pH responses to sequential additions of mitogens in single 3T3 fibroblasts: correlations with DNA synthesis. *J. Biol. Chem.* 263, 11879-11886.

Hunter, T. (1987) A thousand and one protein kinases. *Cell* 50, 823-829.

Kuhn, T. S. (1970): *The Structure of Scientific Revolutions.* The University of Chicago Press, Chicago.

Loeb, J. (1913): *Artificial Parthenogenesis and Fertilization.* Univ. of Chicago Press, Chicago.

Maddox, J. (1988): Finding wood among the trees. *Nature* 333, 11.

Marre, E. (1979): Integration of solute transport in cereals. In *Recent Advances in the Biochemistry of Cereals,* eds. D. L. Laidman and R. G. Wyn Jones, pp. 3-25. New York: Academic Press.

Nelson, N. and L. Taiz (1989): The evolution of H^+-ATPases. *Trends Biochem. Sci.* 14, 113-116.

Ober, S. S. & Pardee, A. B. (1987) Intracellular pH is increased after transformation of chinese hamster embryo fibroblasts. *Proc. Natl. Acad. Sci. USA* 84, 2766-2770.

Oberhaensli, R. D., P. J. Bore, R. P. Rampling, D. Hilton-Jones, L. J. Hands and G. K. Radda (1986): Biochemical investigation of human tumors in vivo with phosphorus-31 magnetic resonance spectroscopy. *The Lancet,* july 5, 8-11.

Perona, R. and Serrano, R. (1988): Increased pH and tumorigenicity of fibroblasts expressing a yeast proton pump. *Nature* 334, 438-440.

Pouyssegur, J., Sardet, C., Franchi, A., L'Allemain, G. and Paris, S. (1984): A specific mutation abolishing Na^+/H^+ antiport activity in harmster fibroblasts precludes growth at neutral and acidic pH. *Proc. Natl. Acad. Sci. USA* 81, 4833-4837.

Pringle, J. R. and L. H. Hartwell (1981): The *Saccharomyces cerevisiae* cell cycle. In *The Molecular Biology of the Yeast Saccharomyces. Life Cycle and Inheritance,* eds. J. N. Strathern, E. W. Jones and J. R. Broach, pp. 97-142. Cold Spring Harbor Laboratory

Raven, J. A. and Smith, F. A. (1976): The evolution of chemiosmotic energy coupling. *J. Theor. Biol.* 57, 301-312.

Serrano, R. (1988): Structure and function of proton translocating ATPase in plasma membranes of plants and fungi. *Biochim. Biophys. Acta* 947, 1-28.

Thomas, R. C. (1989): Bicarbonate and pHi response. *Nature* 337, 601.

Tosteson, D. C. (1964): Regulation of cell volume by sodium and potassium transport. In *The Cellular Functions of Membrane Transport,* ed. J. F. Hoffman, pp. 3-22. Englewood-Cliffs: Prentice-Hall.

Wilson, T. H. and E. C. C. Lin (1980): Evolution of membrane bioenergetics. *J. Supramolec. Struct.* 13, 421-446.

Zetterberg, A. & Engstrom, W. (1981) Mitogenic effect of alkaline pH on quiescent, serum-starved cells. *Proc. Natl. Acad. Sci. USA* 78, 4334-4338.

Hormones and Cell Regulation. N° 14, Eds J. Nunez, J.E. Dumont. Colloque INSERM/J. Libbey Eurotext Ltd. © 1989. Vol. 198, pp. 117-122

Membrane events involved in the action of endothelin and other vasoconstricting hormones

Christian Frelin, Paul Vigne and Catherine Van Renterghem

Centre de Biochimie du CNRS, Parc Valrose, F-06034 Nice Cedex, France

SUMMARY

This chapter defines the relative contributions of the different Ca^{2+} transporting systems when vascular smooth muscle cells are stimulated by the vasoconstrictive peptides : vasopressin, bombesin and the newly discovered peptide endothelin. These are : voltage-dependent and dihydropyridine-sensitive Ca^{2+} channels, receptor-operated non selective channels, Na^+/Ca^{2+} exchange and (Ca^{2+})ATPases of the sarcoplasmic reticulum and of the plasma membrane.

INTRODUCTION

Calcium ions are involved in the regulation of numerous physiological processes. Calcium enters cells either via voltage-dependent Ca^{2+} channels or via yet unidentified receptor-operated channels (ROC). Ca^{2+} may also be released into the cytoplasm by intracellular stores (the sarcoplasmic reticulum in striated muscles and calciosomes) via distinct processes that are mediated by inositol trisphosphate (IP_3) and by Ca^{2+} itself (Ca^{2+}-induced Ca^{2+} release). The mechanisms that decrease the cytosolic Ca^{2+} concentration are the (Ca^{2+})ATPases of the endoplasmic reticulum and of the plasma membrane and the Na^+/Ca^{2+} exchange system (see Carafoli, 1987 for a recent review).

Temporal aspects of variations in the cytosolic Ca^{2+} levels should be important if these variations serve as an intracellular signal for the cells. It is clear that most of the Ca^{2+} that appears in the cytoplasm of vascular smooth muscle cells that are stimulated with vasoconstricting peptides comes from an intracellular pool called calciosomes (Volpe et al., 1988). The role of other Ca^{2+} transporting systems (ROC, voltage-dependent Ca^{2+} channels, the Na^+/Ca^{2+} exchange system and the (Ca^{2+})ATPases of the plasma membrane and of calciosomes) in shaping intracellular Ca^{2+} signals has been less thoroughly analyzed. This chapter defines the relative activities of the different structures in charge of handling Ca^{2+} across the plasma membrane and of calciosomes of aortic smooth muscle cells.

THE VASOCONSTRICTING ACTIONS OF ENDOTHELIN

Endothelin is a newly discovered peptide that is synthesized by the vascular endothelium and that is one of the most potent vasoconstricting substance known so far (Yanagisawa et al., 1988). It acts on aortic smooth muscle cells by activating phospholipase C via a pertussis toxin-insensitive G protein (Resink et al., 1988, Van Renterghem et al., 1988b, Marsden et al., 1989). Membrane inositol phospholipids are hydrolyzed into inositol polyphosphates and diacylglycerol. It is however unlikely that diacylglycerol mediates the contractile action of endothelin, because phorbol esters are poor vasoconstrictors (Forder et al., 1985). IP_3 mobilizes Ca^{2+} from an intracellular pool (Van Renterghem et al., 1988b, Marsden et al., 1989) that is distinct from the caffeine-sensitive pool (Kai et al., 1989). The increase in cytosolic Ca^{2+} level activates a Ca^{2+}-dependent K^+ channel in the plasma membrane and leads to a transient hyperpolarization of the membrane. A partial and transient inhibition of voltage-dependent L-type Ca^{2+} channels is also observed consecutively to the rise in $[Ca^{2+}]_i$ (Van Renterghem et al., 1988a) and to the activation of protein kinase C by diacylglycerol (Galizzi et al.,1987). All these events occured within one to two minutes following the application of endothelin.

A slow depolarization of the plasma membrane due to the opening of a non selective cationic channel that is permeable to Na^+, K^+ and Ca^{2+} accompanies the development of tension. When the membrane potential reaches the threshold potential for the opening of voltage-dependent Ca^{2+} channels, a spontaneous electrical activity develops. Only the latter phase can be blocked by inhibitors of voltage-dependent Ca^{2+} channels (Van Renterghem et al., 1988b).

Thus although a great part of the contractile action of endothelin is prevented by inhibitors of Ca^{2+} channels, the action of the peptide on the Ca^{2+} channel is indirect. Similar findings have been reported for two other vasoconstricting peptides: vasopressin (Van Renterghem et al., 1988a) and bombesin (Lazdunski et al., 1988). One difference is however that endothelin is much less potent than vasopressin (Van Renterghem et al., 1988b) and than angiotensin II (Araki et al., 1989) for stimulating phospholipase C although its contractile activity is larger and longer lasting. It could be that vasoconstriction is not ultimately determined by the extent of the activation of phospholipase C but rather by the opening of the non selective cationic channel of the plasma membrane. One possibility could be that two distinct G proteins mediate the effects of endothelin. One would act on phospholipase C whereas the other would open the non selective cationic channel in the plasma membrane.

ACTIVATION OF Na^+/Ca^{2+} EXCHANGE ACTIVITY BY PROTEIN KINASE C

The properties of the Na^+/Ca^{2+} exchange system in rat aortic smooth muscle cells have been studied using $^{45}Ca^{2+}$ flux experiments and intracellular Ca^{2+} measurements using the dye indicator indo-1 and found to be very similar to those of the cardiac system (Vigne et al., 1988a).

Activation of protein kinase C with phorbol esters increases the activity of the Na^+/Ca^{2+} exchange activity about two-fold. Activation does not result from a change in the membrane potential or of the intracellular Na^+ concentration. Two other important ion transporting systems of the plasma membrane of vascular smooth muscle cells have also been reported to be targets for protein kinase C. Phorbol esters stimulate Na^+/H^+ exchange activity (Vigne et al., 1988c), they partially inhibit voltage-dependent Ca^{2+} channels (Galizzi et al., 1987).

One function of the Na^+/Ca^{2+} exchange system could be to reduce the duration of Ca^{2+} transients induced by Ca^{2+} mobilizing hormones such as epinephrine, angiotensin II, vasopressin and endothelin. Under resting conditions, the transmembrane Na^+ and Ca^{2+} electrochemical gradients are such that the system works as a Ca^{2+} extrusion mechanism (Vigne et al., 1988a). An increase in $[Ca^{2+}]_i$, for instance in response to the mobilization of intracellular Ca^{2+} stores by vasoconstricting peptides, would further promote net Ca^{2+} efflux. Vasoconstricting hormones also activate protein kinase C via the production of diacylglycerol. A protein kinase C-mediated activation of the Na^+/Ca^{2+} exchange system could further promote Ca^{2+} efflux and reduce the duration of Ca^{2+} transients. To test this hypothesis, Ca^{2+} transients were induced by vasopressin in smooth muscle cells under conditions in which the Na^+/Ca^{2+} exchange system was forced to function as a Ca^{2+} influx mechanism or was rendered inactive by depleting cells of their Na^+. In all cases the Ca^{2+} transients had the same size and time course as those elicited in cells that have a Na^+/Ca^{2+} exchange system that operated as a Ca^{2+} efflux mechanism. Similar results have been obtained for angiotensin II-induced Ca^{2+} transients. These experiments indicate that the Na^+/Ca^{2+} exchange system is not involved in the short-term regulation of cytosolic Ca^{2+} levels of aortic smooth muscle cells and that this function is mainly achieved by the (Ca^{2+})ATPases of the calciosomes and of the plasma membrane. The Na^+/Ca^{2+} exchange system could be involved in the long-term maintenance of intracellular Ca^{2+} levels. The same function has been postulated for the system in cardiac cells (Carafoli, 1987).

THE PLASMA MEMBRANE CONTROLS THE CALCIUM LOAD OF CALCIOSOMES

Vasopressin and bombesin activate phospholipase C in aortic smooth muscle cells and produce large and similar intracellular Ca^{2+} transients that reach a maximum at 10 seconds and decrease to resting level within 2 minutes. Ca^{2+} transients are independent of the presence of extracellular Ca^{2+} and resulted from the mobilization of intracellular Ca^{2+} stores. Only half of Ca^{2+} that is released into the cytoplasm after hormonal stimulation is pumped back into calciosomes and can be mobilized in response to the application of a second peptide. The remaining Ca^{2+} is pumped outside of the cells (Doyle and Ruegg, 1985; Vigne et al., 1988b). Calciosomes were depleted of their Ca^{2+} by a 1-2 hour exposure of the cells to a 50 nM Ca^{2+} medium. Depletion occured faster at 4°C than at 25°C. Upon shifting Ca^{2+}-depleted cells to a Ca^{2+}-containing medium, intracellular calcium stores refilled slowly ($t_{1/2}$ = 4 minutes). (−)D888, a blocker of voltage-dependent Ca^{2+} channels, and Ni^{2+}, a putative blocker of receptor-operated Ca^{2+} channels (Hallam and Rink, 1985) slowed the kinetic of refilling of calciosomes. These experiments indicate that the rate limiting step for refilling calciosomes once Ca^{2+} had been mobilized by IP_3, is Ca^{2+} influx through the plasma membrane. This was demonstrated in a more direct way by showing that if Ca^{2+} uptake by the Na^+/Ca^{2+} exchange system is promoted, then calciosomes refill almost instantaneously (Vigne et al., 1988b). A refilling of calciosomes from the extracellular space as described for acinar cells (Merritt and Rink, 1987) was not observed in aortic smooth muscle cells (Vigne et al., 1988b). It seems therefore that Ca^{2+} efflux out of the cells via the (Ca^{2+})ATPase serves to desensitize vascular smooth muscle cells to the repetitive actions of different vasoconstricting peptide. In addition, one role for voltage-dependent Ca^{2+} channels (and for the electrical activity of the plasma membrane) could be to control the importance of the Ca^{2+} stores and therefore to control the responsiveness of the cells to the action of circulating peptides. A similar function has been suggested for Ca^{2+} channels (Morad and Cleeman, 1987).

Acknowledgements

This work was supported by the "Centre National de la Recherche Scientifique", the "Association pour la Recherche contre le Cancer" and the "Fondation sur les Maladies Vasculaires". We are grateful to M.-T. Ravier, N. Boyer and C. Roulinat-Bettelheim for expert technical assistance and to Dr. J.-P. Breittmayer for flow cytometic analyses.

REFERENCES

Araki, S., Kawahara, Y., Kariya, K., Sunako, M., Fukuzaki, H., and Takai, Y. (1989): Stimulation of phospholipase C mediated hydrolysis of phosphoinositides by endothelin in cultured rabbit aortic smooth muscle cells. Biochem. Biophys. Res. Commun. 159:1072-1079.

Carafoli, E. (1987): Intracellular calcium homeostasis. Annu. Rev. Biochem. 56:395-433.

Doyle, V., and Ruegg, U.T. (1985): Vasopressin induced production of inositol trisphosphate and calcium efflux in a smooth muscle cell line. Biochem. Biophys. Res. Commun. 131:469-476.

Forder, J., Scriabine, A., and Rasmussen, H. (1985): Plasma membrane calcium flux, protein kinase C activation and smooth muscle contraction. J. Pharmacol. Exptl. Ther. 235:267-273.

Galizzi, J.P., Qar, J., Van Renterghem, C., Fosset, M., and Lazdunski, M. (1987): Regulation of calcium channels in aortic muscle cells by protein kinase C activators (diacylglycerol and phorbol esters) and peptides (vasopressin and bombesin) that stimulate phosphoinositide breakdown. J. Biol. Chem. 262:6947-6950.

Hallam, T.J., and Rink,T. (1985): Agonists stimulate divalent cation channels in the plasma membrane of human platelets. FEBS Letters 186:175-179.

Kai, H., Kanaide, H., and Nakamura, M. (1989): Endothelin sensitive intracellular Ca^{2+} store overlaps with caffeine sensitive one in rat aortic smooth muscle cells in primary cultures. Biochem. Biophys. Res. Commun. 158:235-243.

Lazdunski, M., Romey, G., and Van Renterghem, C. (1988): Bombesin modulates the spontaneous electrical activity of rat aortic cells (A7r5 cell line) by an action on three different types of ionic channels. J. Physiol. (London) 407:100P.

Marsden, P.A., Danthuluri, N.R., Brenner, B.M., Ballermann, B.J., and Brock, T.A. (1989): Endothelin action on vascular smooth muscle involves inositol trisphosphate and calcium mobilization. Biochem. Biophys. Res. Commun. 158:86-93.

Merritt, J.E., and Rink, T.J. (1987): Regulation of cytosolic free calcium in fura-2 loaded rat parotid acinar cells. J. Biol. Chem. 262:17362-17369.

Morad, M., and Cleeman, L. (1987): Role of Ca^{2+} channel in development of tension in heart muscle. J. Mol. Cell. Cardiol. 19:527-553.

Resink, T.J., Scott-Burden, T., and Buhler, F.R. (1988): Endothelin stimulates phospholipase C in cultured vascular smooth muscle cells. Biochem. Biophys. Res. Commun. 157:1360-1368.

Van Renterghem, C., Romey, G., and Lazdunski, M. (1988a): Vasopressin modulates the spontaneous electrical activity in aortic cells (line A7r5) by acting on three different types of ionic channels. Proc. Natl. Acad. Sci. USA 85:9365-9369.

Van Renterghem, C., Vigne, P., Barhanin, J., Schmid-Alliana, A., Frelin, C., and Lazdunski, M. (1988b): Molecular mechanism of action of the vasoconstrictor peptide endothelin. Biochem. Biophys. Res. Commun. 157:977-985.

Vigne, P., Breittmayer, J.-P., Duval, D., Frelin, C., and Lazdunski, M. (1988a): The Na^+/Ca^{2+} antiporter in aortic smooth muscle cells. Characterization and demonstration of an activation by phorbol esters. J. Biol. Chem. 263:8078-8083.

Vigne, P., Breittmayer, J.-P., Lazdunski, M., and Frelin, C. (1988b): The regulation of the cytoplasmic-free Ca^{2+} concentration in aortic smooth muscle cells (A7r5 line) after stimulation by vasopressin and bombesin. Eur. J. Biochem. 176:47-52.

Vigne, P., Breittmayer, J.-P., Frelin, C., and Lazdunski, M. (1988c): Dual control of the intracellular pH in aortic smooth muscle cells by a cAMP-sensitive HCO_3^-/Cl^- antiporter and a protein kinase C-sensitive Na^+/H^+ antiporter. J. Biol. Chem. 263:18023-18029.

Volpe, P., Krause, K.H., Hashimoto, S., Zorzato, F., Pozzan, T., Meldolesi, J., and Lew, D.P. (1988): Calciosomes, a cytoplasmic organelle: The inositol 1,4,5-trisphosphate-sensitive Ca2+ store of non muscle cells? Proc. Natl. Acad. Sci. USA 85:1091-1095.

Yanagisawa, M., Kurihara, H., Kimura, S., Tomobe, Y., Kobayashi, M., Mitsui, Y., Yazaki, Y., Goto, K., and Masaki, T. (1988): A novel potent vasoconstrictor peptide produced by vascular endothelial cells. Nature 332:411-415.

RESUME

Ce chapitre définit l'importance des contributions relatives des différents systèmes de transport de Ca^{2+} lorsque des cellules de muscle lisse vasculaire sont exposées à des peptides vasoconstricteurs : vasopressine, bombésine et endothéline. Ces différents systèmes sont : les canaux Ca^{2+} dépendant du voltage et sensibles aux dihydropyridines, les canaux non sélectifs activables directement par les récepteurs membranaires aux peptides, l'échangeur Na^{+}/Ca^{2+} et les (Ca^{2+})ATPases du réticulum sarcoplasmique et de la membrane plasmique.

Colloques **INSERM**
ISSN 0768-3154

Other *Colloques* published as co-editions by John Libbey Eurotext and INSERM

153 Hormones and Cell Regulation (11th European Symposium). *Hormones et Régulation Cellulaire (11ᵉ Symposium Européen)*.
Edited by J. Nunez and J.E. Dumont.
ISBN : John Libbey Eurotext 0 86196 104 8
INSERM 2 85598 324 X

158 Biochemistry and Physiopathology of Platelet Membrane. *Biochimie et Physiopathologie de la Membrane Plaquettaire*.
Edited by G. Marguerie and R.F.A. Zwaal.
ISBN : John Libbey Eurotext 0 86196 114 5
INSERM 2 85598 345 2

162 The Inhibitors of Hematopoiesis. *Les Inhibiteurs de l'Hématopoïèse*.
Edited by A. Najman, M. Guigon, N.-C. Gorin and J.-Y. Mary.
ISBN : John Libbey Eurotext 0 86196 125 0
INSERM 2 85598 340 1

164 Liver Cells and Drugs. *Cellules Hépatiques et Médicaments*.
Edited by A. Guillouzo.
ISBN : John Libbey Eurotext 0 86196 128 5
INSERM 2 85598 341 X

165 Hormones and Cell Regulation (12th European Symposium). *Hormones et Régulation Cellulaire (12ᵉ Symposium Européen)*.
Edited by J. Nunez, J.E. Dumont and E. Carafoli.
ISBN : John Libbey Eurotext 0 86196 133 1
INSERM 2 85598 347 9

167 Sleep Disorders and Respiration. *Les Evénements Respiratoires du Sommeil*.
Edited by P. Lévi-Valensi and D. Duron.
ISBN : John Libbey Eurotext 0 86196 127 7
INSERM 2 85598 344 4

169 Neo-Adjuvant Chemotherapy. *Chimiothérapie Néo-Adjuvante*.
Edited by C. Jacquillat, M. Weil, D. Khayat.
ISBN : John Libbey Eurotext 0 86196 150 1
INSERM 2 85598 349 5

171 Structure and Functions of the Cytoskeleton. *La Structure et les Fonctions du Cytosquelette*.
Edited by B.A.F. Rousset.
ISBN : John Libbey Eurotext 0 86196 149 8
INSERM 2 85598 351 7

Colloques **INSERM**
ISSN 0768-3154

172 The Langerhans Cell. *La Cellule de Langerhans.*
Edited by J. Thivolet, D. Schmitt.
ISBN : John Libbey Eurotext 0 86196 181 1
INSERM 2 85598 352 5

173 Cellular and Molecular Aspects of Glucuronida-
tion. *Aspects Cellulaires et Moléculaires de la Glucu-
ronoconjugaison.*
Edited BY G. Siest, J. Magdalou, B. Burchell
ISBN : John Libbey Eurotext 0 86196 182 X
INSERM 2 85598 353 3

174 Second Forum on Peptides. *Deuxième Forum
Peptides.*
Edited by A. Aubry, M. Marraud, B. Vitoux
ISBN : John Libbey Eurotext 0 86196 151 X
INSERM 2 85598 354 1

176 Hormones and Cell Regulation (13th European
Symposium). *Hormones et Régulation Cellulaire (13ᵉ
Symposium Européen).*
Edited by J. Nunez, J.E. Dumont, R. Denton
ISBN : John Libbey Eurotext 0 86196 183 8
INSERM 2 85598 356 8

179 Lymphokine Receptors Interactions. *Interactions
Lymphokines-récepteurs.*
Edited by D. Fradelizi, J. Bertoglio
ISBN : John Libbey Eurotext 0 86196 148 X
INSERM 2 85598 359 2

191 Anticancer Drugs (1ˢᵗ International Interface of
Clinical and Laboratory responses to anticancer
drugs. *Médicaments anticancéreux (1ʳᵉ Confrontation
internationale des réponses cliniques et expérimenta-
les aux médicaments anticancéreux).*
Edited by H. Tapiero, J. Robert, T.J. Lampidis
ISBN : John Libbey Eurotext 0 86196 223 0
INSERM 2 85598 393 2

193 Living in the Cold (2ⁿᵈ International Symposium).
La Vie au Froid (2ᵉ Symposium International).
Edited by A. Malan, B. Canguilhem
ISBN : John Libbey Eurotext 0 86196 234 9
INSERM 2 85598 395 9

Reproduction photomécanique
IMPRIMERIE LOUIS-JEAN
BP 87 — 05002 GAP
Tél. : 92.51.35.23
Dépôt légal :611 — Septembre 1989
Imprimé en France